GW00417578

THE woman BOOK OF

Beauty and Health

Other *Woman* Books

The Best of *Woman* Fashion Knitting
The Best of *Woman* Family Cooking
The *Woman* A–Z of Family Health
Actionwoman's A–Z of Consumer Rights

Vickie Bramwell

THE
woman
BOOK OF

Beauty and Health

GRAFTON BOOKS

A Division of the Collins Publishing Group

LONDON GLASGOW
TORONTO SYDNEY AUCKLAND

Grafton Books
A Division of the Collins Publishing Group
8 Grafton Street, London W1X 3LA

Published by Grafton Books 1988

British Library Cataloguing in Publication Data

Bramwell, Vickie
  The Woman book of beauty and health.
  1. Women. Health – For women   2. Women.
  Beauty care – Manuals
  I. Title
  613′.04244

ISBN 0-246-13194-2

Printed in Spain by
Cronion S.A., 08004 Barcelona

Contents

This book is dedicated to my husband, Nick Brookes

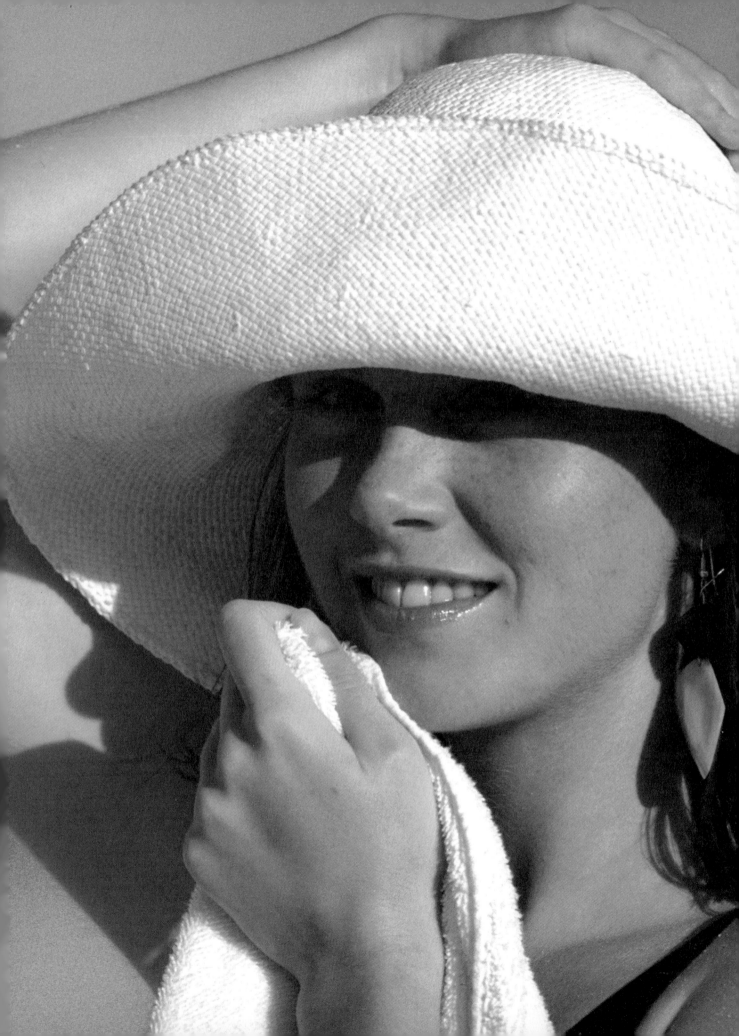

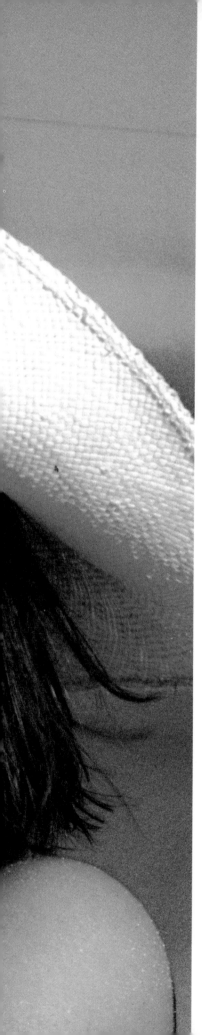

Introduction

There's a lot of nonsense talked about beauty. This beauty book isn't going to add to it. The aim is to give you practical and enjoyable information which will help you look, and feel, better. I believe in knowing the basics. You can then find a style and fitness plan to suit you.

Looking after your skin and body makes sense. The better you treat them the better and longer they'll serve you. Good health and fitness improve the quality of life – just think about aching feet as an example of how to ruin an occasion! In fact, fitness contributes to appearance (imagine your face with those sore feet), and appearance does matter – it's the first thing you're judged by. Research has shown that you have about ten minutes after meeting someone to alter or crystallise their idea of you from the initial visual impression. You can have fun with that first impression if you like: make-up, perfume and hairstyle, along with clothes, can create a visual image that you'd like to give, be it businesswoman, outdoor type or unadorned innocent. But no great shadow is going to fall across your path if you go out bare-faced. You should use make-up if or when it suits *you* rather than because you feel you ought. Some women (and I can imagine my predecessors in the beauty business having vapours) look and feel better without it.

What's more important is the level of happiness and contentment you're feeling, and that is always reflected in your face and posture. Beauty can help you with this through health – as I've mentioned – and self-confidence built by a well-toned, clean look that we call attractiveness. I've never come across a woman without the potential for beauty but I've seen plenty who haven't realised it properly.

And that's what I hope this book will do – help you to use your body and image to their best advantage. More than all that, I hope you have fun in the process.

CHAPTER 1

An Application to Beauty

Beauty isn't just for the beautiful. But it does take some strategy to make the best of your appearance and style.

The first basic on the beauty trail is to get to know your good and bad points so that you can make the most of the good ones and treat – while playing down – the bad ones. You don't have as many occasions to 'see' yourself as the world does: three dimensionally, in different lights, as make-up wears off or skin gets drier or grimier after a long day. So give yourself the best basis for beauty treatment by making a personal study of yourself.

Get to know your outer covering. The best way to assess your skin type is without make-up and in daylight. Notice if your skin is

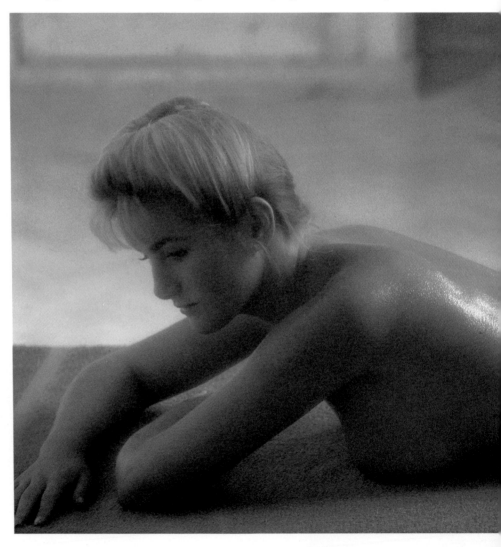

dry, flaky, greasy or blemished. Do you have broken veins? Is it dull and sallow, flushed and high-coloured? Use two mirrors to examine your facial skin side view. Take notice of skin at your hairline or sides of nose; under your chin, the parts you don't usually see. Write down how your skin is and read Chapter 2 for everything you need to know on how to condition it to look and feel soft and smooth.

Hair is one of the first things that people notice about you, but how often do you look at your hair from the back and side view or notice how the roots look from the top or at a side parting? In daylight again, take notes on the condition of your crowning glory: is

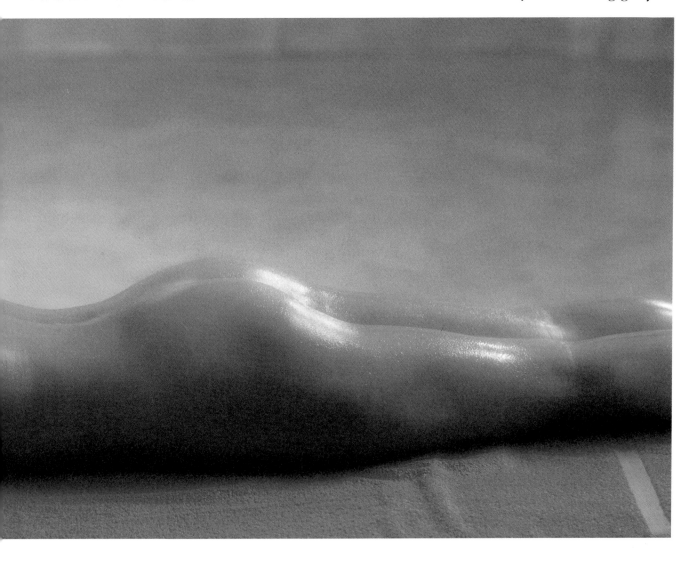

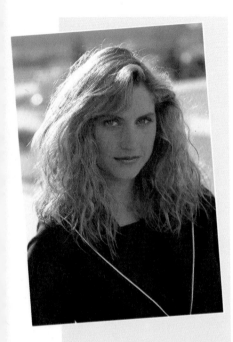

it dry, greasy, split at the ends, too thin, too thick? Do you have a flaking scalp? Visualise a different style to flatter your face shape; take it off or pull it onto your face to see how it suits you. Armed with this information, Chapter 3 gives you a complete guide on how to get your hair into top condition, change its look and find a hairdresser for personal advice on cut, colour and curl.

Flatter yourself and have fun with colour. Whether you like using make-up discreetly or boldly, always or just for special occasions, there's an art to how you put it on. The right applicators, shades and types of products for your colouring and for the situation in which you're wearing it make all the difference between make-up using you or you using make-up! Chapter 4 has the foundations for a perfect make-up look plus more information for those who wish to make up different looks for different occasions.

Finding your own style is probably the trickiest and most enjoyable part of beauty, as we're all so different. Chapter 5 won't do it for you but it will point you in the right direction. And remember that your individual style will change as you progress from young and lovely to older and sophisticated. So if you feel you need an update, this will help you too.

A good figure can give you confidence and make you look lithe and lively. An immediate improvement may be correcting posture (which takes a few minutes) or a spot of exercise to firm up certain areas (which takes a little longer). And if you'd like to be a few pounds lighter, try this test: look at yourself with nothing on in front of a full-length mirror. Now lift your arms above your head and stand on tiptoe. This is how you'd look around half a stone lighter. While you're there, notice your side and back view, too. Note the areas you need to work on to get into good shape. Chapter 6 will tell you how to get the best looking body.

Making your body beautiful means being nice to know with careful hygiene, a fresh or scented smell and smooth silky body skin. Not damaging your skin by careless sunbathing is the best way to keep it looking younger. Find out how to keep your body smooth, soft and sweet in Chapter 7.

Hands, legs, feet and bottoms are our supporting features. They work harder than the rest of you and can therefore suffer from the effects of friction or pressure. The special beauty care these extreme assets need is detailed in Chapter 8 and will help them provide you with good looks and longer service.

Good health is a must for beautiful looks. Taking care of your teeth and sight, the right to change a feature that you consider ugly and sorting out health problems which affect a woman's delicate make-up, should be a part of every woman's beauty routine. Chapter 9 is a rundown on all the things that may run you down!

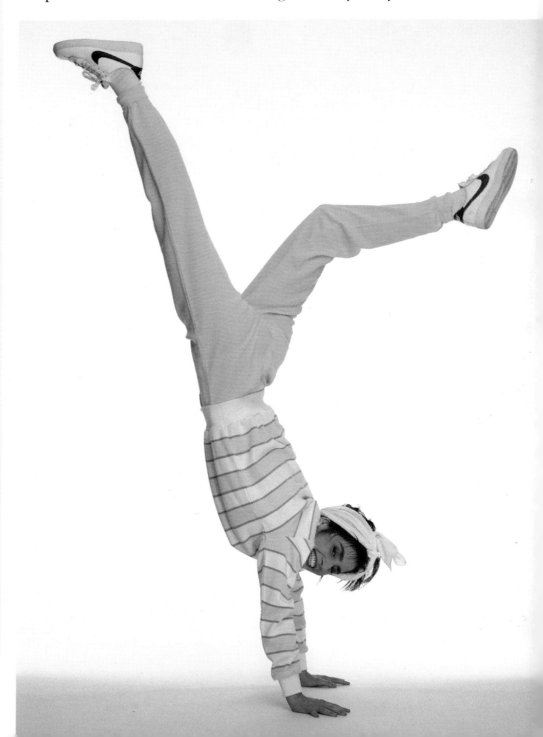

Relaxation and energy are what keep you looking your best. With the inner beauty treatments in Chapter 10, you'll be lovely to look at and to know: avoiding stress, calming down and boosting energy for when you need it.

Beauty salons/ health clubs

These offer a wealth of services and treatments to soothe and smooth you. Whether you go regularly or once in a blue moon for a treat, the aim is relaxation while experts help to make you look and feel more beautiful. Beauty salons, clinics or health clubs/farms should always be clean, dry and warm. The staff here should inspire confidence with a pleasant, helpful manner and not try to press you into treatments that you don't want. Always ask for the full price before booking a treatment and ask the receptionist if tips are appropriate and, if so, how much they should be. If you feel that a salon or club doesn't come up to standard, complain loudly to the manager or owner. If you think it's dirty or damp, do everyone a favour and report the salon to the local trading standards authority or council who give them their trading licence. Failing that, write and suggest an exposé to the local newspaper!

Many of the treatments offered at beauty salons or health clubs can be done yourself, at home (plenty are outlined in this book), or you may wish to see how an expert beautician does it before trying a treatment at home (for example a facial or make-up). Some treatments should only be carried out by experts. Below is a rundown of what you may find on your local salon's menu!

Facials are cleansing and relaxing treatments with cleansers, masks, often steam treatments to relax pores, toners and massage. Iontophoresis treatments use an applied electrical current at a safe strength and aim to stimulate circulation, cause perspiration and relax pores. Specially prepared products are said to help the electrical current draw impurities from the skin. Galvanic masks are a rubbery solution, left on the face for around 20 minutes with an electrical current applied for extra impact. Cathiodermie uses a galvanic current, then an emulsion covered by gauze and massaged with high frequency electrodes; this is followed by a massage to tighten pores again.

Body massages and aromatherapy aim to tone up the body with

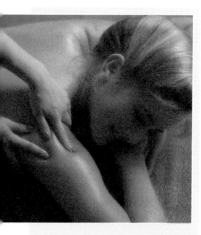

massage using oils or lotions. In the case of aromatherapy, the added oils treat other ailments by smell or, enthusiasts believe, essences sinking into the skin – though there's no scientific proof that this can happen.

Electrical massage, with pads wired to a safe electrical current either strapped on or applied by a masseur, aims to cause the muscles to relax and contract, stimulate circulation and help tone up stubborn fatty areas. A tingling sensation is usual but some find these treatments too vigorous.

Saunas, steam cabinets and Turkish baths all aim to use heat and steam to produce water loss through perspiration. Apart from weight loss, which is easily replaced when you rehydrate yourself by drinking, they're also said to rid toxins from the body through sweat.

Reflexology is an ancient Oriental art and type of foot massage which is said to release hidden obstacles blocking the body's energy lines and causing bodily ills.

Waxing, either hot or 'cool' (which is in fact, warm), removes superfluous hair on the body. A waxy solution (although some are now honey-based) is applied to the skin and then ripped off bringing hairs with it. Comments on pain vary from 'discomfort' to 'agony'.

Diathermy aims to seal off red thread veins or recurring spots. Electrical current passes down a fine needle which singes the capillary. As there is a danger of scarring through unskilled operation, this should *only* be done by a qualified beautician who has at least five years' training in electrolysis.

Electrolysis. Electrical current is applied through a fine needle to an individual hair root to destroy it. The same rules apply as for diathermy; this should only be attempted on the face by a qualified beautician with at least five years' experience. Both of these electrical treatments often take more than one session to work permanently.

OTHER TREATMENTS

Many of these are considered to be alternatives to conventional medicine. Some are practised in health clubs or farms along with beauty treatments or you may find experts with individual practices. These healing processes can be used together with other therapies or on their own, either to fight a specific symptom or to keep the body generally healthy.

Holistic medicine starts by assessing the total character and tries to cure ills by using a combination of alternative medicines to treat the whole person, thereby tackling an illness at source rather than simply treating symptoms.

Homoeopathy uses herbs and mineral remedies to create symptoms similar to the one that the body is fighting in an effort to build up immunity and treat the mental attitude. Homoeopathy is sometimes used with conventional medicine for on-going disabling diseases.

A career in beauty

Beauticians (either specialised in one subject or with varied experience) are found in most high street department stores, health clubs, leisure salons, clinics and sometimes larger hotels and hairdressers, too. If you feel that you'd like to get into the beauty business, think carefully about what is involved. Although the job appears glamorous, you'll have to be prepared to take the less glamorous side, too. You'll need to be genuinely interested in people and possess a sympathetic nature; tact, patience and discipline are the basis of a successful career. A beauty treatment such as waxing superfluous hair or a body massage puts your client in a vulnerable position; you'll be expected to help her relax as part of the job.

If you're not sure, a spell of part-time work in a beauty clinic will give you some understanding of what is required. Training in basic anatomy, physiology (especially of the skin) and the various treatments is vital. Your town hall or local library may be able to help by giving you details of courses available. Or for a career booklet, syllabus and list of schools, send a stamped addressed envelope to The British Association of Beauty Therapy and Cosmetology, Suite 5, Wolseley House, Oriel Road, Cheltenham, Glos GL50 1TH.

Skincare companies sometimes give training to their own beauty consultants. Ask one of the consultants at a large store or beauty salon how you could go about being accepted for training.

Make-up artists for photographic, TV or film work usually begin by training as beauticians. Some, including top make-up artist Barbara Daly, began their careers in the make-up department of a television company. Others start as hairdressers and, after creating hairstyles for photography and film for some time, pick up enough tips on make-up to start doing the make-up artist's job, too.

Beauty journalists usually get a basic journalistic training (often on a local newspaper) before specialising in beauty. Others discover that they have a talent for writing while working within the beauty industry (in Public Relations, for cosmetic companies, for example) and then make the transition to beauty writer.

Anyone choosing a beauty career must be interested and ready to get involved with other people. They must care about how people feel and look as the beauty business isn't only concerned with outward appearance but also with how we feel about ourselves.

CHAPTER 2

Skin and Sensibility

Skin is the body's packaging. It keeps harmful elements out and vital body fluids in. But it does much more than that.

Although waterproof on the outside, skin allows water and waste products out and, through shivering and sweat, regulates temperature. Perspiration is a mixture of water, fatty acid and bacteria, and we sweat between one and twenty pints or between a half and twelve litres of it a day. Not only does this lubricate and seal in the skin's moisture but it also helps repel harmful germs and bacteria. Skin is more elastic than rubber and, if healthy, will easily shrink to fit substantial weight loss or expand to accommodate weight gain. Skin gives us the preventative and pleasurable sense of touch. Containing 70 per cent water, it is the largest organ of the body, covering around 17 square feet/2 square metres and weighing around 7lb/3k for the average person.

Skin is the outside image that you show the world. Soft, glowing, umblemished skin is as much a beauty plus as bright eyes, shiny hair or a healthy figure. But, luckily, those who haven't got a good complexion can work hard at making it better, while disguising it when necessary by taking advantage of the many products specially designed for the purpose on the market today.

The state of your skin is similar to your temperament – it owes a lot to your parents but it also reflects what has happened to you since you were born. Skin will show up what's going on inside your body – illness, hormonal imbalances (puberty, pre-menstruation, pregnancy, menopause) or stress may affect the condition short-term. Prolonged bad diet, stress, lack of moisture (dry atmosphere, dehydration), some drugs and ultraviolet light (from sun and sunbeds) will damage the condition long term. What you are, what you do and what you eat are reflected in this most effective body covering. And if it breaks down or deteriorates towards later life, not only your looks but your health can suffer as a result. Skin is worth looking after.

What is skin?

The cleverest of scientists or engineers could not have designed it better. The three layers which basically constitute skin all play a complicated and vital role in its effectiveness and appearance.

The lower layer (sub-cutis or hypodermis), houses fat cells, tissue and blood vessels which feed and pad the upper layers.

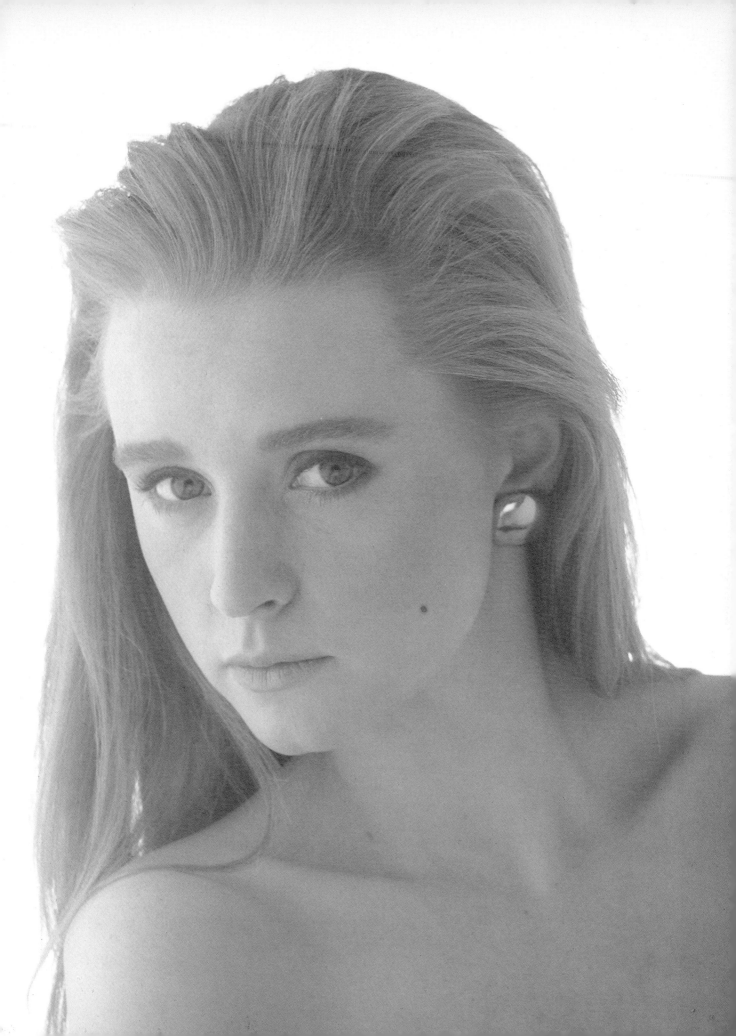

The middle layer is called the dermis and it's this layer which when it breaks down will do most harm to the skin's overall condition. The dermis contains elastin and collagen fibres in a gel type of substance which together act as a kind of springy mattress to the skin, giving it firmness, bounce and elasticity. Also in the dermis are blood vessels which give skin its pinky glow, nerve endings, sweat glands and hair follicles with pores.

Between the dermis and epidermis (the top layer of dead skin cells that we see) is the basal layer. The basal layer holds a kind of blueprint system for skin cells, constantly manufacturing new upwardly mobile ones in a 28-day cycle through the epidermis. The epidermis also contains melanocytes, which form pigment, naturally or through ultraviolet exposure. Under a microscope, surface skin cells are similar to fish scales, overlapping each other like tiles. These top cells flake off constantly (in dry skin, you can see it happening) leaving healthier newer cells underneath and preventing the build-up of a dead, dull covering.

How to have soft, glowing skin

Apart from taking preventative action against ageing (see Ageing Skin section), you can help keep your skin healthy by cleansing regularly to remove dead skin cells, sweat and oil, and by making sure that the moisture level is kept up.

All skin types and both sexes should clean skin twice a day. The most convenient time is morning, to remove the night's debris (skin cell growth is faster while you sleep), and last thing at night to remove the dirt and grime of the day.

While applying a water and oil mix (lotion or cream) on your skin helps put and keep some moisture in, drinking enough liquid is just as important. Skin gets most of its moisture from the inside, as moisturisers can't sink into the dermal layer. Four pints/2 litres of water a day is ideal (more on hot days or in dry atmospheres) – and remember that foods such as salads can contain up to 96 per cent water.

CLEANSING

Water alone is not enough and won't dissolve oil-based make-up or sebum, the skin's natural oil. Ninety-seven per cent of women in

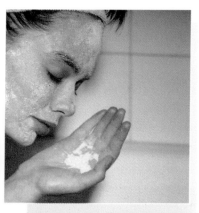

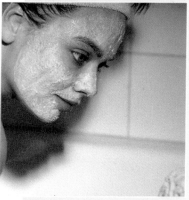

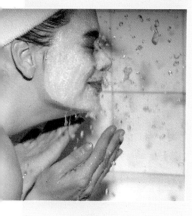

Britain use a cleanser or cold cream on their faces – it should be 100 per cent – and that includes men, too. The alternatives are a rinse-off or tissue-off cleansing product.

Rinse off

Soap is a cleanser but is alkaline-based so can strip your mainly acid-based skin of too many of its natural oils. While removing the grimy sebum, you want to retain the skin's natural acid mantle which acts as protection to keep it waterproof, while housing bacteria to protect skin from infection. Harsh detergent (as in soap) will dry out and break down fine facial skin's top layers. While many still believe in the old soap and water routine (and it certainly beats nothing at all), it's not recommended if your skin is very dry or sensitive (see chart on p. 16). And if you must use soap on your face, aim for an unperfumed brand, rinse thoroughly with lukewarm water and moisturise quickly afterwards.

A *cleansing bar* (or soapless soap) looks and performs like a soap but is pH acid/alkali balanced to match your skin, so doesn't trigger the degenerative effects. Cleansing bars come in all shapes and forms and usually lather less than soap (you don't *need* lather for cleansing – boosters are added by manufacturers, along with perfume and colour, because we like them).

Wash-off or rinsable cleansers should be applied to skin with clean fingertips in circular motions and splash-rinsed off with tepid water. They are ideal for those who like the fresh feel of water on their face. And remember to wash your flannel, if you use one, after every use.

Tissue-off

Cleansing milks and lotions are oil-in-water formulations which are lighter than creams and should be applied with fingertips or cotton wool, using dabbing motions, to take away the grime. Some of these can wash off, too – try a damp cotton wool pad or splashing with lukewarm water.

Cleansing creams are thicker water-in-oil emulsions suitable for heavy make-up removal or drier skin. They should be massaged on to the skin in gentle, circular motions with fingertips; then tissued off. You'll need to use a toner to remove residue.

Toners dissolve the last greasy residue of cleansers and leave skin feeling cool – but do avoid eyes and dilute the toner if you've sensitive or dry skin. They aren't needed if you use a rinse-off cleanser.

Eye make-up removers are special in that they're unperfumed and less clogging to the eyes while being specially effective in dissolving waterproof mascaras. Best application to this delicate area is gently, with clean fingertips. Remove thoroughly with short strokes of a soft tissue – cotton wool can leave filaments in the eyes. Splash eyes with cold water to remove residue after use.

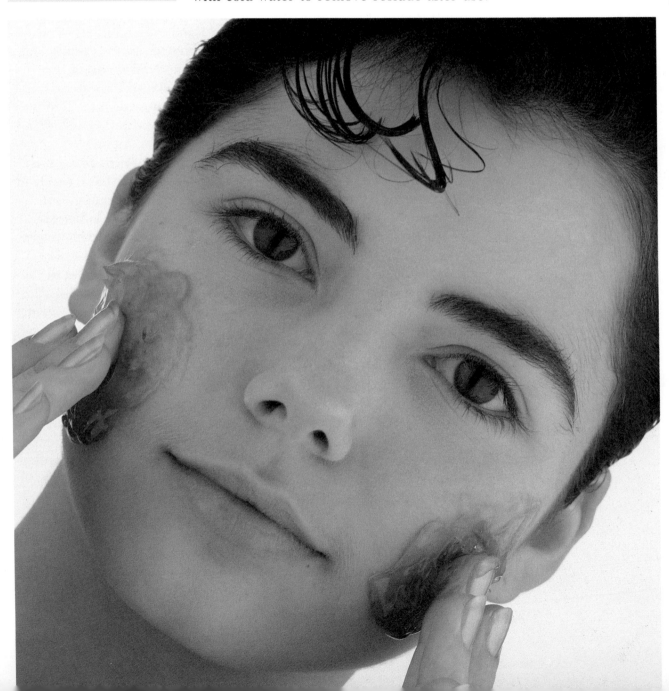

Face masks can be deeper cleansing, dermabrasive (removing top layer of dead skin cells), hydrating or anti-bacterial (for spots). Read the instructions carefully to find the right one for you – and don't use more than once a week on dry or sensitive skins.

MOISTURISERS

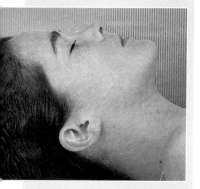

Loss of water by illness or an arid atmosphere creates dehydrated skin which looks rough and flaky. Dehydrated skin can allow damaging outside influences to penetrate, making it feel sore and irritable. The main function of a moisturiser is to add and seal in water. As already mentioned, the skin is continuously pumping out sebum – a mixture of water and oil (fatty acids) with bacteria and waste products. One of the functions of sebum is to act as a natural moisturiser for lubrication, smoothing and sealing the skin's surface. Combined with cleansing – to remove stale sebum and the build-up of the dirt it attracts – moisturiser reinforces this action.

Some moisturisers include other claims such as 'nourishing' and 'anti-ageing'. Some claim to sink down to the basal (living) layer and help protect and speed production of skin cells. Others list ingredients found in the skin such as lipodeac acid and collagen. Whether most of these claims are justified is still being argued over by dermatologists and really not relevant to healthy younger skin (for older skin, see Ageing Skin section). The only added ingredient that's recommended in a moisturiser is a sunscreen (against ultraviolet light), so seek out these by reading the pack information or leaflets carefully.

What's a moisturiser? The answer is: anything that's oily and waterproof (and that includes margarine or cooking oil – but these don't feel pleasant to the skin). Purpose-made skin moisturisers are devised to sink into the surface skin cells and feel silky, while not smelling too bad. Most moisturisers, like make-up and washing powder, have added perfume. It seems that the great British public prefer to have scent in their skincare even though it is more likely to produce an allergic reaction and certainly doesn't help the skin. Unfragranced, unperfumed and hypo-allergenic products do not smell of anything. Use your sense of smell to find out if moisturisers are scented.

There are two basic types of moisturiser on the market: the first is a lighter and thinner oil-in-water emulsion which contains up to 80 per cent water; these are therefore more liquid and sink in or

	TEST	CLEANSER	TONER	MOISTURISER
Dry	Flakes easily Feels taut Rarely shines	Cream or lotion	Mild or diluted	Three times a day, after cleansing and midday
Sensitive	Easily gets blemishes Easily irritated by sun, wind, polluted atmospheres, illness and some drugs Sometimes gets allergies	Hypo-allergenic or unperfumed	Hypo-allergenic or unperfumed	Hypo-allergenic or unperfumed Twice or three times a day according to dryness
Combination	Greasy panel of concentrated sebum glands down forehead, nose, central cheeks and chin (Try tissue pressed against nose – grease leaves mark)	As for dry and greasy in relevant areas	Only with non-rinsable cleansers	As for dry and greasy on relevant sections
Normal	Neither taut and flaky nor greasy and shiny Behaves well	Any of the range	Yes – with cream and lotion No with rinsable cleanser	Twice a day after cleansing
Greasy	Shines, tissue shows marks	Cleansing bar or rinsable	No	Light moisturiser twice a day

SKIN TYPE

evaporate quickly. Lighter moisturisers often contain humectants (honey, glycerine and so on) which attract water from the air in humid atmospheres. The problem with these is that in dry atmospheres (weather, central heating) they'll take water from the nearest source and that could be the skin – so beware where and when you use them. Water-in-oil moisturisers are better for drier skins or atmospheres as they're thicker, creamier and, although they take some time to sink in, give a good sealing layer. You can generally tell which category a moisturiser is in by the look and feel but the distinctions are becoming blurred with advanced formulations – usually the thicker and more solid, the more oil they contain and the better for older, drier skin or dehydrating atmospheres.

For problem, extra dry skin (damaged and flaking), a good way of making sure you're adding water and keeping it there, is to put on a humectant light moisturiser and follow it with a creamier thick one. But be sure you've worked out your skin type correctly – too heavy moisturising can clog pores and lead to water retention and puffiness, especially overnight when activity is slower and the body more sluggish. If this happens with your normal moisturiser, consider a slightly thinner consistency. Moisturiser is best applied to slightly damp, warm skin. Wait at least half an hour to allow it to sink in before putting on make-up.

Eye creams are lighter moisturisers for use on the delicate, fine skin around the eye area. Heavier lotions can clog and create puffiness. They are often gels.

Necks. Ascertain your neck skin type (which may vary from your face) and cleanse, tone and moisturise as facial skin.

Ageing skin

'Nature determines the face you have at 20. Your lifestyle determines the face you have at 30. At 50 you have the face you deserve.'

These are the immortal words of Coco Chanel. But is it true that if you nurture your skin with the latest anti-ageing products, old age will repay you with a smooth, younger-than-your-years complexion?

Certainly some of the manufacturers who are currently flooding the market with 'miracle' hydrating, anti-wrinkle and assorted regeneration preparations would have us believe they do.

HOW DOES SKIN AGE?

The way skin ages is said to be determined by your genes and sex, but these in turn are governed by age and affected by the care you've taken as well as by the environment. The epidermis (top layer) and the dermis (lower layer) become thinner as you get older, sometimes to the point of transparency so that underlying veins become visible. This is due to skin functions slowing down and becoming less efficient with age. Elastin and collagen production, which maintain firmness and elasticity, slow down; skin cells don't retain moisture so well and become flatter quicker but are shed and renewed more slowly. Sebum production slows down, causing drier skin. Wrinkles form where collagen and elastin beneath have been imprinted by facial muscle actions such as smiling and squinting.

But you can help to slow down the ageing skin process by taking some sensible measures. The damage caused by UVA and UVB rays (see Suntanning Section, Chapter 7) is said to be the single greatest external cause of ageing. A prime trigger of collagen and elastin breakdown, sunlight also promotes 'free radicals'. These highly charged chemicals are said to be activated and become aggressive in response to injury (including UV light). They cruise the bloodstream and, if not mopped up by enzymes, can launch an attack on the cell nuclei and blueprint for new cell growth (DNA). Once a cell is deformed, it may not be able to reproduce efficient and effective new cells. UV light can do damage at any age and so determine the rate and degree of ageing – not to mention the risk of skin cancer. But you can protect yourself from further damage whatever age you are. Avoid sunburn at all costs by going out protected in intense sun or always wearing a foundation in which the pigment acts as a sunscreen.

Moisturise. Older skins take on a sagging, rough and flaky appearance. The rigorous use of a moisturiser, applied often, helps to plump up surface cells and seal in natural moisture, helping older skin, in particular, to look firmer. Dermatologists say that only the fine skin lines caused by excessive dryness are masked by moisturising creams. Many of the 'anti-wrinkle' creams fall into this 'moisturiser' category – 'super' hydrating creams which plump up the surface skin cells.

It is when moisturisers are called 'anti-ageing', 'rejuvenating', 'nourishing', 'regenerating' that the debate starts. Can a cream's

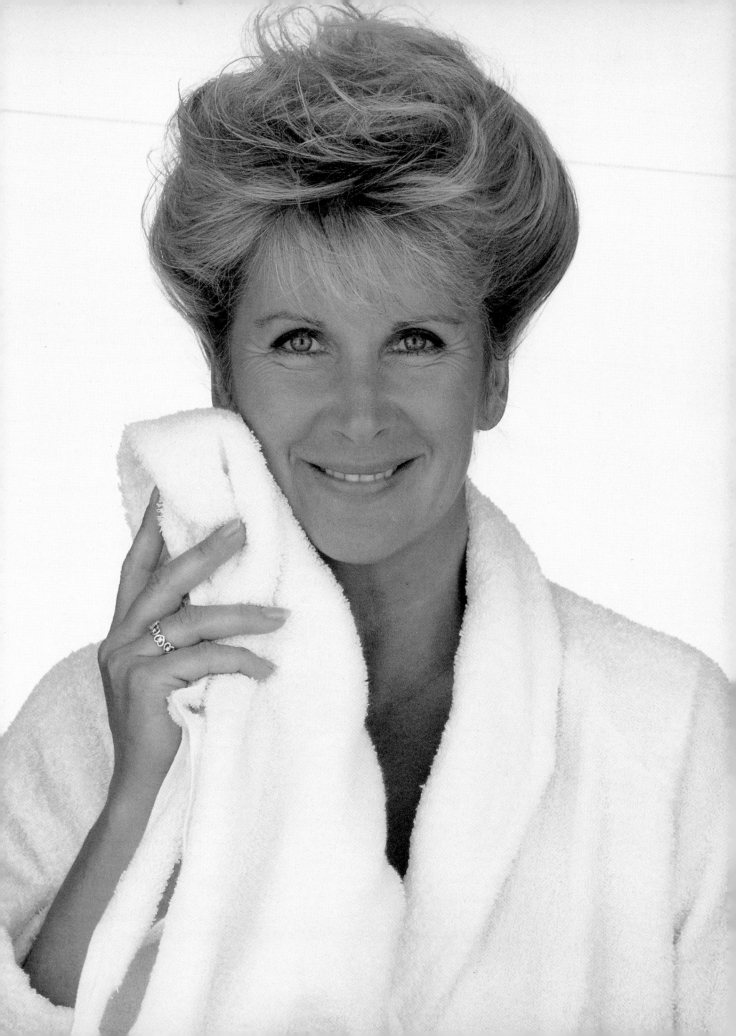

THE WOMAN BOOK OF
BEAUTY AND HEALTH

20

'active' ingredients penetrate beyond the epidermis and help *living* cells work more effectively, as some of the products aimed at older skins claim?

Some manufacturers would have us believe that ingredients in their serums penetrate the lower skin layers and push the production of new cells into overtime or reinforce the skin's renewal system of supporting collagen and elastin fibres. But many dermatologists argue that the skin's function is to provide a barrier and that these creams and lotions can *only* be absorbed by the uppermost layer of dead cells, where they act like any other moisturiser.

Most 'anti-ageing' miracle ingredients contain molecules which are far too big to get below the skin's surface layers when applied on top. Collagen and elastin, although found in the skin, are two such substances.

But a few chemicals have proved to be able to reach the dermis and get into the bloodstream; it's whether they do any good when they get there that is open to debate.

'To expect a foreign protein to go through the epidermis and align itself in structure and function to the body's tissue fibres is similar to trying to restore the stability of a rusting, unsafe iron bridge by dropping nuts and bolts on it,' said one leading dermatologist.

The only creams guaranteed to deliver are those used medically (such as steroids put on the skin's surface). In Britain, anything which penetrates the top layer of skin to the dermis is considered pharmaceutical, not cosmetic, but the distinction has become very narrow.

So-called 'repair' serums give instant extra plumpness to the skin's surface and could make facial lines appear less deeply etched simply by over-saturating and sometimes stretching the skin. These products can inflame sensitive skin, too.

The latest miracle ingredients are called liposomes – tiny spheres of phosphorus and fats which can be 'loaded' with chemicals and aimed at skin cells. Liposomes *can* actually do some good when used medically, for other purposes, but whether the ones used in skin creams break up before or fuse with cell membranes when they get there is still arguable. And can a liposome cargo significantly influence an ageing cell? The debate continues. Linoleic, or fatty, acids are thought to nurture cell growth and development. But scepticism about how they work in skin creams is rife.

In fact, whether any of these anti-ageing and anti-wrinkle creams work will only be revealed as today's generation of users reach old age. One thing is sure, though, the search for eternal youth will continue. And also do remember that any benefits will only last as long as you use the product. If it feels good, use it but don't expect miracles; and do continue to invest only in products that give results which you can see and feel.

The following may also help to keep skin younger for longer:

Exercise. Regular exercise leads to muscle tone and a sense of well-being which is reflected in your skin. Fresh air brings life to a dull complexion.

Relaxation. Stress and anxiety can give a careworn appearance to the skin, as your body takes from cell renewal to cope with the anxiety. Frowning and taut facial muscles cause wrinkles. Adopt a relaxation technique (see Chapter 10).

Avoid smoking and drinking. Apart from the obvious health risks, smoking can increase the development of facial lines and can deprive skin of the nutrition it needs. Excessive drinking can deplete the body's supply of vitamins C and B and dehydrate the skin.

Watch your diet. Keep your weight down and you'll look younger. But don't go on starvation or crash diets as these deplete the body and collapse the fat needed for firmness on the face because ageing skin isn't capable of readjusting its elasticity easily. Crash diets will also deprive the skin renewal process of the nutrition it needs to function. Be sure you're getting an adequate balanced diet and drinking plenty of water as skin is hydrated from inside, too. If you need to, lose weight slowly and healthily (see Shape up, Chapter 6).

Skin problems

Contrary to what most of the skincare companies seem to think, spots don't always magically disappear when you're out of your teens. Often it's more like the mid-thirties, sometimes even later. Skin blemishes from boils to blackheads, acne to allergy can occur to anyone at any age. Here are some suggestions on knocking them out.

Acne. Believed to be hormonal and genetic in origin, acne can be devastating to anyone but is doubly hard on teenagers who are going through many types of change due to hormonal activity. Boys often suffer from acne vulgaris (or teenage acne) more than girls owing to the androgen hormone. Acne rosacea (red acne and not related to the teenage type) usually develops later in life and is aggravated by sunlight, heat, stress and spicy foods.

Acne occurs when skin cells start to overproduce and the sebaceous (oil) glands become blocked by clumps of dead skin, hindering the free flow of sebum and resulting in infection. Stress can trigger a worse attack, so although it's easy to say and hard to do – don't panic. Teenage acne does disappear, usually in the early twenties, sometimes later; meanwhile, try to lessen the effects. Don't over-stimulate the skin with strong skincare for greasy skin or use abrasive treatments – they will over-stimulate the oil glands and worsen the problem. Instead, use a specially prepared benzoyl peroxide treatment from your chemist to unplug skin pores and help fight infection. Use it once a day and then try to leave skin well alone. A doctor may prescribe antibiotics (these sometimes interfere with the Pill and pregnancy – check). Your doctor may also consider hormone treatment tablets (similar to the Pill with the same side-effects and only suitable for women) or a relatively new drug called Roaccutane, derived from vitamin A and successful in treating acne although there can be side-effects. It should only be given by a specialist and not taken if there's a possibility of pregnancy.

Finally, remember not to pick or squeeze spots, scarring will remain when the acne has gone. If you're unlucky enough to be scarred, zyderm collagen injections can fill out some of the pits but this is a costly and lengthy business and needs to be topped up every 6 to 12 months (see Cosmetic Surgery section in Chapter 9).

Rashes: allergy and skin irritation. Eczema and contact dermatitis come under these banners but any irritation, whether just in one place or all over, with itching, redness, a rash, bumps or flaking, can be an allergic or irritant reaction. If you're a hayfever, asthma or migraine sufferer, you're more likely to get allergic skin reactions and in extreme cases they can be life threatening. Irritant reactions are less severe and only occur at the site of contact (e.g. hands with washing-up liquid). Rashes can be caused by an outside influence (metal, sunlight) or an internal one (strawberries, penicillin).

You *can* be allergic to anything – even, in some very rare cases, to water. However, in skincare, rashes are mainly caused by lanolin, perfume or preservatives. Allergy can be alleviated by anti-histamine tablets and in some more dangerous cases a drug to speed up

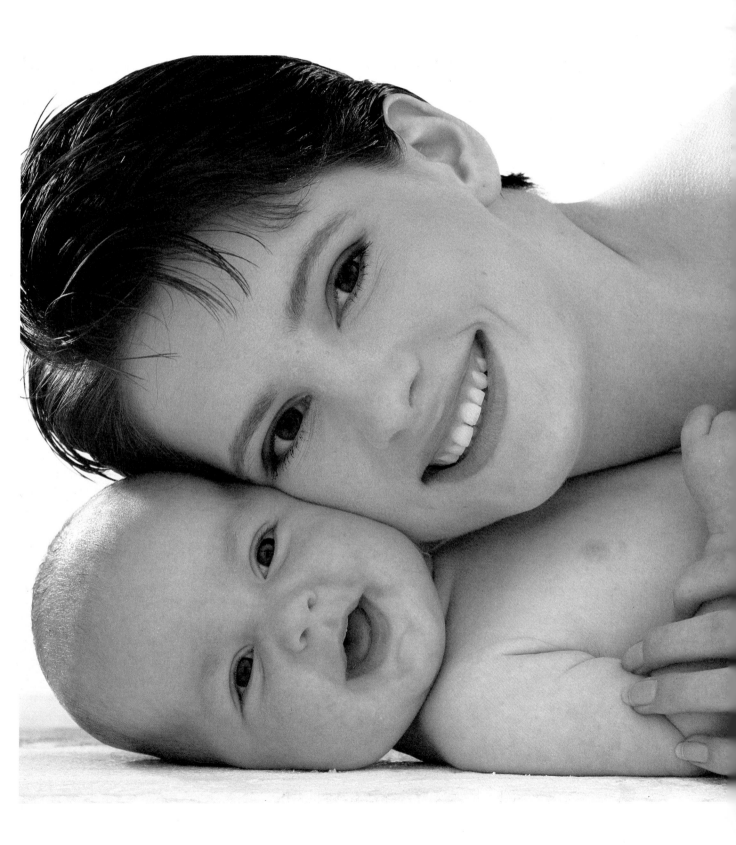

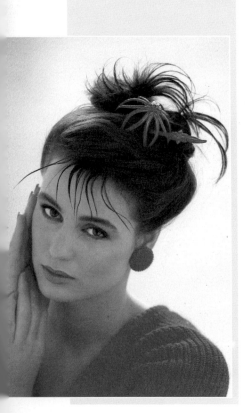

metabolism and remove the allergen from the body faster. Cortisone cream and lotions can soothe and protect the area but by far the best treatment is to find the culprit. Most skincare products labelled hypo-allergenic have passed a test for the absence of well-known allergens and irritants. But that's not to say you won't be affected by them and it's best to try a dab, rubbed into your inside elbow or wrist, for 24 hours before buying. Remember also, if you're prone to rashes, to wear cotton-lined rubber gloves for housework and use fragrance-free soaps for bathing.

Blackheads are nothing to do with dirt. They're plugged pores where dead surface skin and sebum have been trapped. Deposits of melanin (the pigment that is responsible for suntanning) and oxygen in the air turns the pore black. Unfortunately those with a greasy skin or greasy panel on their face are more prone to open pores and blackheads. The best way to prevent them forming is by scrupulous cleansing with an oil-free cleanser to remove dead surface skin. Weekly face masks or very gentle sloughing with granular sloughing creams will help unblock pores.

Boils. Unpleasant and painful, boils result from bacterial infection in blocked pores or from ingrown hairs and can strike especially when you're run down, under stress or have recently been ill. A magnesium sulphate paste from your chemist will help 'draw' the boil. In bad cases, your doctor may lance it and/or give you antibiotics.

Cold sores are caused by a virus called herpes simplex which hibernates in the skin until triggered into action, usually by extreme cold or heat during periods of stress. They are contagious so beware of sharing towels or flannels and don't touch them unless necessary – then wash your hands before touching other areas of your (or someone else's) skin. A chemist can give you lotions to soothe the sores or your doctor may prescribe an anti-viral drug. If you're a regular sufferer, wear strong sunblocks over the area in hot climates, as UV light may provoke attacks.

Moles. Clumps of natural pigment (like permanent freckles), moles are usually harmless. If a mole starts changing shape or colour, begins to bleed, becomes painful or suddenly appears, consult your doctor immediately. Malignant melanoma is a particularly deadly skin cancer and on the increase in Britain owing to our sunbathing habits. But this type of pigmental cancer is curable if caught early enough. Never try to remove a mole yourself and seek your doctor's advice if you have one in a place where it's constantly rubbed (e.g. by a bra strap or when combing your hair). Check moles regularly for changes in appearance.

Rough skin patches. A skin patch which won't heal and looks rough and sore should be checked by a dermatologist – go to your doctor for a referral. Skin cancer is probably the most simple carcinoma to detect and cure.

Whiteheads occur when bacteria attack the accumulated sebum in a blocked oil duct. This causes redness and swelling, so the body reacts by attracting millions of white blood cells to combat the inflamed area and a spot forms. They can be treated with a drying, antiseptic lotion from the chemist.

Cysts are a harmless build-up of dead skin and a blocked oil gland which doesn't become inflamed. They can be removed by a dermatologist, if you wish.

Warts. Like cold sores, warts are caused by a dormant and contagious virus promoting a build-up of rough skin. Sometimes they will just disappear; sometimes they'll suddenly appear in later life. While the acid solutions available from the chemist, which slowly dissolve the wart, are fine for hands and feet (verrucae), they should not be used on the face. See a dermatologist instead.

Broken veins are caused by ruptured blood vessels – mainly in skin thinning through heredity, age, steroid treatment, too much sun, alcohol or high blood pressure. A covering make-up base can disguise them. Electrolysis or sclerotherapy (where a chemical is injected) can seal fine thread veins and capillaries around the face (see Hair Removal section, Chapter 7 and Cosmetic Surgery, Chapter 8) but your operator should be a member of the Association or Institute of Electrolysists and have been practising for at least five years. Laser treatment or sclerotherapy to close the vein are available from dermatologists and cosmetic surgeons.

Pigmentation patching. See Suntanning section, Chapter 7.

Psoriasis. This rapid scaling and flaking of skin which can affect people for years, or just occasionally, is still largely a mystery but is thought to be hereditary. It can come in patches or all over the body. If you suspect that you're a sufferer, visit your doctor for consultation and prescribed treatment.

Vitiligo. These white patches on the skin (the opposite to freckles) which show up more with tanning are usually just a quirk of nature; there is no cure. Protect these areas from the sun as there is a lack of melanin there to protect them, and cover them with a foundation or fake tan if you feel they look unsightly.

What does it mean?

Here's a run-down on all those scientific sounding, on-pack ingredients in skincare:

Allergens. Ingredients which have been known to trigger an allergic response.

Collagen. A protein in the dermis which gives structure, softness and suppleness to the skin. Although it does break down in the skin when damaged or ageing, collagen in skin creams can't replace it.

DNA. Deoxyribonucleic acid – the molecules which contain the genetic material or blueprint for the life of the cell. It includes information on how the cell functions.

Exfoliation. A process which strips away the surface layer of dead skin cells. The aim is to prevent build-up and dryness while allowing new softer skin to show through. You can achieve this by sloughing with a soft brush or cream containing granules which is

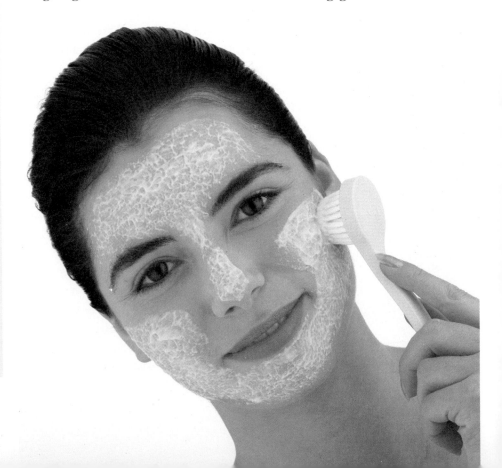

massaged over the skin and then rinsed or tissued off.

Free radicals. Electrically charged unstable particles which can damage the DNA or enzymes in the skin when motivated in response to injury, such as UV light. Whether creams or pills can prevent their doing damage is open to question.

Hypo-allergenic. A product which is less likely to produce an allergic reaction. It will have been formulated without and/or tested against well-known allergens. Most hypo-allergenic products are perfume-free but many contain preservatives.

Melanin. The brown pigment contained in most skins (albinos are the exception) which is encouraged to appear as a tan by the sun's rays. Its function is to help protect the skin from burning.

Non-comedogenic. Comedo is a blackhead, genic means 'make them'. A non-comedogenic skincare product is not oily and so won't clog pores.

Nourishing. A widely misused word in skincare. These creams imply that they impart more than moisture to the skin. Many dermatologists still believe that only water can effectively help dry or ageing skin.

pH. The surface skin's acid/alkaline balance; an average person has around 5.5 acid to 4.5 alkali.

Photosensitivity. A reaction triggered by sunlight on skin, often showing up as redness. May be caused by perfume in skincare.

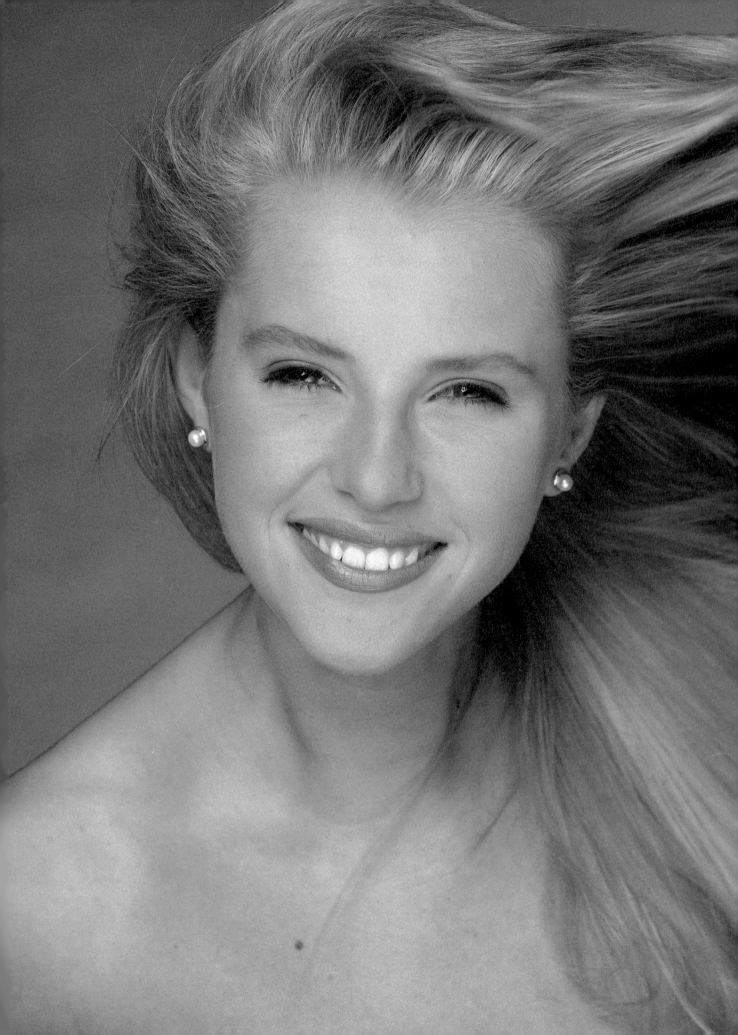

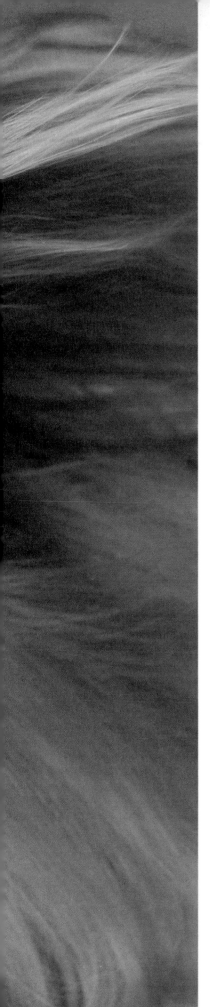

CHAPTER 3

Hair, Hair

The average person has between 100,000 and 150,000 hairs on their head at any one time. Blondes have the highest number, followed by brunettes, with redheads having the fewest. These hairs are a hangover from prehistoric times when hair served the purpose of protecting us from cold and abrasion. Today, hair is one of the first things that people notice about you and in a crowd it distinguishes you from others. Hair is also one of the natural beauty assets that takes minimum effort to use to your best advantage. The beauty of hair is that it is so changeable – in just a couple of hours you can switch your shade to a blonde bombshell, ravishing redhead or sultry brunette. In a few minutes, with the array of popular products on the market, you can become a mass of curls, straight and sexy, make hair into a shining dressed style or wide volumed and wild. Like fashion, hair is there to be used to suit your personality, whim and mood. And luckily – because hair does take a beating from dyeing, perming, relaxing and overheating – it keeps on growing, so is constantly renewed. Having said that, you need to look after your hair to get the best from it, especially the roots, which give a constant supply of more.

Hair is basically dead protein, in a slightly different form from our nails. The roots (living part) are joined to nerves, sebum glands and the blood supply to keep producing healthy new hair. But abuse the ends and they'll stay damaged; there are no warning devices or nutritional supplies there to reinforce or repair, which is why damaged, longer hair needs conditioners to do the work instead. Each hair has its own cycle length (usually 1–6 years) and grows at the rate of about half an inch every month (more in hot weather). You lose between 100 and 150 hairs every day. New hairs are growing all the time. An unhealthy diet, illness, stress or trauma can affect new hair growth at the root. So if hair is weakened at this point you may find it breaks off more easily later (at, say, one inch of growth from the scalp) when you have forgotten about the original cause. This shows how important it is to keep hair roots healthy. Apart from a healthy blood supply with plenty of oxygen and nutrients, the scalp also needs to be kept clean, moisturised and unclogged for good hair growth and to allow the hair's natural protective oil, sebum, to escape and coat the hair.

Hair problems

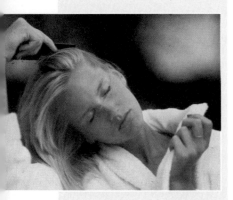

Baldness, when hair falls out from the roots, is often hereditary at a certain age in men, less frequently in women. Unfortunately, there is no proven cure. Twelve per cent of men under 25 suffer from it and 45 per cent under 45. Research male ancestors to find out the likelihood in your family. Baldness can also be caused by hormonal upset (post-pregnancy, the Pill), shock, some drugs, X-ray, overprocessing (bleaching, perming), gland disorders, imbalances in nutrition or over-enthusiastic hairstyling. If necessary visit your GP for referral to a trichologist or dermatologist.

Psoriasis and eczema are often hereditary but are aggravated by allergy or stress. The characteristic scaly skin may form on other parts of the body, too. Visit your GP.

Dandruff is often just a dry scalp (in the same way as dry skin occurs on other parts of the body) or flaking from deposits left by shampoo, conditioner or mousse from the hair rather than the scalp. Other forms of scaliness caused by infection, often accompanied by greasiness and/or itching and sometimes baldness, are caused by a variety of conditions from hormonal upheaval (for instance, at puberty) to lack of some vitamins and stress. See your GP.

Head lice or nits are itchy parasites with no regard to social status or cleanliness. They're very contagious and if one person in the family has them, the whole family should be treated as soon as possible. Treatment from your GP is quick and effective.

Greasy hair shows most on fine hair. Regular, gentle shampooing keeps the scalp clean. Too much heat (from heated appliances such as hairdryers) will over-activate the sebum gland and cause oilier hair.

Dry hair will benefit from scalp massages and brushing hair often to push sebum glands into more action. Dryness may also be caused by overprocessing the hair (by colour or curl products) or by a dry environment. Add and seal in moisture with hair conditioners.

Hair care

Clean hair. Contrary to past opinion, washing your hair as frequently as you'd like to won't damage it – if you do it properly. Just like skin, hair benefits from regular cleansing to remove dirt and debris (old skin cells from the scalp), and as clean, sweet-smelling hair is nice to know, it's worth doing as often as once

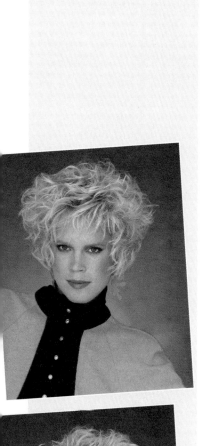

a day if time permits. But there is a right and wrong way to go about it.

Here's the right way: first brush hair and massage scalp to loosen dead scales and release any flaky residue of mousse, gel or spray. Now, using running water (a hand-held or fixed shower, as bath water is already dirty if you're in it), dampen hair through, without soaking it. Always use warm water for washing and rinsing; too hot and it dries out the scalp and damages the hair, too cold and the shampoo won't work effectively. Always use mild shampoo on chemically treated hair, as some anti-dandruff formulations can fade coloured and dry, permed hair. Pour the shampoo on to the palm of one hand to cover the area of a 50p piece and smooth it over both palms, then over hair from the crown backwards. If your hair is very long or thick, it's worth taking the shampoo on to your fingertips and dabbing it at the roots along partings over your head, to make sure you get more even distribution. If it's very greasy, apply mild shampoo directly to dry roots and then add water. Now massage the shampoo in with your fingertips (this is a good time to give yourself a good head massage to boost circulation at hair roots). Make sure you use the pads of your fingers rather than your nails for massage to avoid breaking the hair or scratching your scalp.

Massage for at least two minutes, then rinse under running water for at least two minutes (time yourself if you're not sure). As some scalp problems and dandruff-type conditions stem from residue of detergent (which is what shampoo basically is), it's important to rinse it all off for a healthy head. Conditioner can be smoothed on to just the ends (if scalp is oily) or all over (if scalp is dry). Gently comb it through for even distribution and leave conditioner on for the recommended time – as they vary in strength and holding power you may find that they wash off completely if you rinse too soon, and make hair floppy and sticky if you leave them on too long. Now rinse again for two to three minutes (longer on long, thick hair) and, if you're brave, finish off with a cold rinse to help flatten hair cuticles. Pat hair dry with a towel rather than rubbing it, which can cause breakage to wet, vulnerable hair. The kindest way to dry hair is naturally but this isn't often practical; so pat it towel-dry first then dry while styling with the coolest heat on your dryer.

Glossy hair. If hair is extra dry or has been chemically processed (with colorants, permanent curl or relaxing products), you'll need extra conditioning. To be effective, these hairdressing techniques

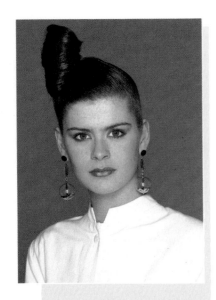

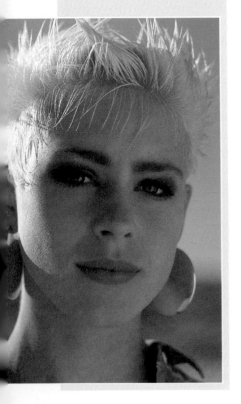

require the hair to be changed inside the hair shaft. There are many, many products on the market to condition hair but the most efficient way is with the aid of heat to help open the tiny hair cuticles (the 'pores' which when seen under a microscope overlap like fish scales). These are usually slightly open and roughened when hair is damaged by dryness or hairdressing treatments. Conditioner, like moisturiser, sinks into the hair through the cuticle and helps to stick them down again – producing a smoother, shiny look. The best way to add heat to a conditioning treatment at home is to wrap your head in a towel, cling film or tinfoil after applying it. However silly it looks, your head's natural heat then helps the conditioner sink in, while not drying it out too quickly. Another way is to condition hair the night before you wash it, allowing it to dry and stay on the hair for a few hours before washing out.

Brush it beautifully. Brushing longer, wet hair with a bristle brush will stretch and damage it. Use a bristle brush, instead, to brush between washes and help to distribute scalp oil along the hair shaft. Special brushes with rounded spike ends are made for wet hair – or use a comb with blunt-ended teeth. Start at the ends and work upwards to avoid pulling and breaking from tangles.

Setting products have recently flooded the market and revolutionised at-home styling. Mousse gives volume and strong hold to hair sets while not being as rigid as hairspray. Use it on towel-dried hair (water dilutes and won't give such good holding power). 'Conditioning' mousses have the added advantage of avoiding hair getting over-dry and prevent some of the flaking often mistaken for dandruff. Gels are extra strong and come in wet or dry finished looks to help style smoother hair shapes or stick them up in a spiky style. Setting sprays and the like give an extra strong finishing hold and are used in the same way as hairspray, to add strength to a set; some are more flexible and less rigid than others – read the labels. If your hair begins to look dull and dry, it could be that you're not washing and rinsing it thoroughly enough to remove these products from your hair; a little residue each time will build up and not allow your natural shine to show through.

Hair in the sun. Just like skin, hair can be broken down and damaged in harsh sunlight. Although more mousses and conditioners now contain sunscreens, they're not usually strong enough to give protection on an all-day sunbathing session on holiday. A hat or scarf will stop ultraviolet rays reaching inside your hair's shafts and breaking the sulphur bonds – it's this that weakens hair and fades colour resulting in frizzy, dry, unmanageable locks.

Hair in the water. Salt in the sea or chlorine in the pool can damage hair, too. Either keep it out of the water (put it up or wear a cap), rinse with clear water afterwards (take a bottle to the beach, most pools have clear water showers around them) or apply conditioner beforehand to protect it.

All about hairdressers

Hairdressers in Britain are known the world over for being the best and most creative. You'll find British hairdressers in the most far-flung corners of the globe and overseas hairdressing students flock to Britain for information and inspiration. Teasy Weasy, Vidal Sassoon and, more recently, Trevor Sorbie and John Frieda are all British hairdressers known internationally. Can you think of any foreign ones? Yet still we moan. Like the good old British GP, communication between public and professional hairdresser breaks down frequently. Why?

Hair, like dress, is a fashion item, and we treat it like one: changing shape and style regularly. The difference is that we can't take hair off if we no longer like it or discover that it doesn't suit us. And, in the case of hairdressing, it requires someone else to be totally responsible for the look. With clothes, it's our responsibility: we try them on, decide to buy them and then either choose to wear them or not. With hair, we might have all the same aspirations as with fashion: renaissance look (with long flowing curls), a geometric bob (shining angular cuts), a Farrah Fawcett or Princess Diana style. We like the look and go to the hairdresser's to 'buy' it.

This may give your hairdresser a problem. A good one will recognise what you are trying to achieve (so far so good) but often the hair isn't the right texture, colour, condition and so on; and your face may be a different shape so the end result won't look like the ideal. Your hairdresser has two options: to try to achieve a close enough, possibly impractical style which may not suit you or refuse to do it. A good hairdressing client will appreciate the honesty and, if she is not able to see it for herself, ask another hairdresser for a second opinion. A bad hairdresser who does the impractical, unflattering style, or an unreasonable client who doesn't see why it

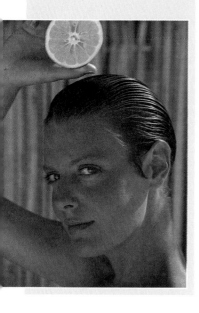

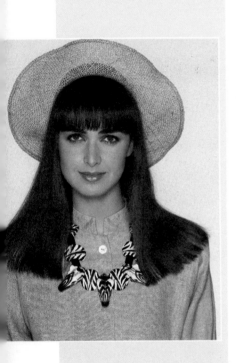

shouldn't be done, provide most of the hairdressing problems around.

A degree of trust is needed. A good, reputable hairdresser will give a free consultation and be happy for you to go away and think about it before booking an appointment. After all, it's in their interests for you to become a contented regular customer and for them to gain a good local reputation. You should never be pressurised into extra treatments (and that includes conditioning treatments) without having a chance to think about them. And you have reason to complain loudly and to the owner if the towels or combs used aren't clean (please *do* complain for the sake of the next unsuspecting client, even if you have vowed never to go back). Don't put up with harsh treatment of your hair; if it hurts or is breaking off, stop them doing it. And don't sit there silently while a 'washer' is not watching what s/he is doing.

Things that make life difficult for a hairdresser, apart from clients who insist on impractical styles, are people who forget to mention in booking that they'd like a perm or colour (if you're kept waiting, this is usually the reason); people who change their minds half way through a perm or colour (it's impossible to stop the process completely); those who don't mention that they're pregnant, taking drugs or have been ill (which can affect hair condition and sometimes means that certain treatments are not recommended), or who complain about the bill (work out how much the average hairdresser must earn after spending an hour or more on your hair, then deduct costs for heating, lighting, electricity, rent and rates).

So by stating clearly what you like and don't like, while discussing what is possible, appropriate and flattering to your hair, communication between hairdressers and clients may get better. And if you've found a hairdresser who suits you – hang on to him or her! It's going to be a fruitful friendship for both of you.

Complaints about your hairdresser or salon? First go back to the salon and consult the owner/manager. If s/he is unhelpful, you can take legal advice: you can claim for personal injury although you'll need a medical report and photographs of the injury. But be warned – it can get complicated and expensive by the time your case is heard. It could be easier and quicker to accept compensation from the salon.

Perming

Today's perms are more versatile than ever, so if you never ate your greens and have straight hair but long for gentle waves or even a bit of bounce; perming is the answer.

The word 'perm' is short for permanent wave. Hair is wound on rollers, then chemicals are applied to open the cuticles and soften the sulphur bonds so making it flexible. After being left to develop, sometimes with heat, a neutraliser stops the chemical action and allows the new shape to set.

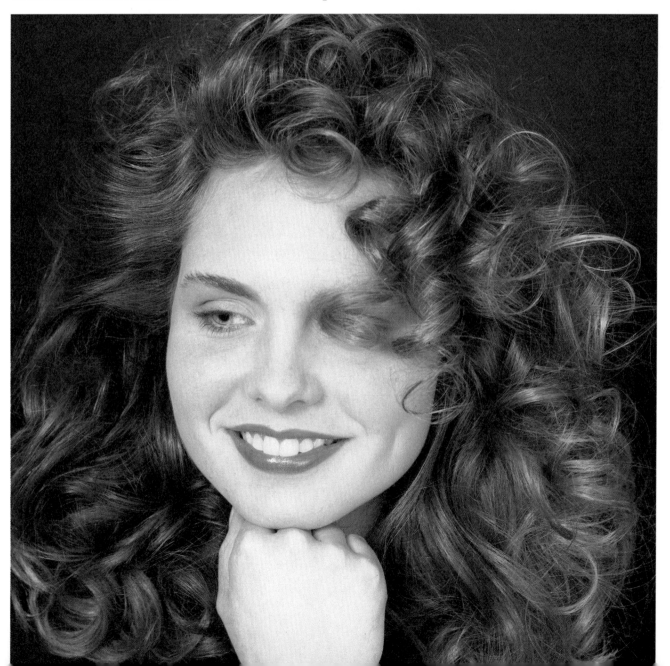

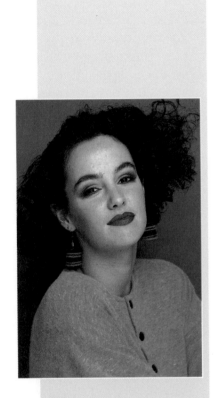

Don't consider a home perm if your hair is already damaged or coloured. Some home perms are gentle enough to use on slightly damaged or carefully coloured hair but these hair types are best left to a hairdresser's expert advice.

If you decide to perm, try the style you're aiming for by curling it first to decide whether you like it enough to wear it permanently. Ask your hairdresser to do this if you're going to a salon. Hair should be permed before colouring, as perming chemicals can strip hair colour. It's wise to have your cut after a perm so it can accommodate and flatter the new style. Short hair *must* be cut afterwards to allow enough hair to wind effectively round a roller for the perm.

At home. Choose a perm that suits you. Find the right size rollers for your hair length and the style you wish to achieve. All home perm products show styling techniques in their leaflets, but basically the smaller the rollers, the tighter the curl. If hair is not in tip-top condition, you'll find the perm takes more easily and you'll get a tighter look in shorter time, but you'll also find that hair looks even more damaged. Do an allergy and curl test 24 hours before perming (a strand at the nape of the neck is best, so that it's covered by outer hair). If you decide to go ahead, ask a friend to help with the back rollers which you won't be able to reach so well. Follow pack instructions to the letter. And do make sure you cover rollers completely with perm solution and neutraliser to get an even look.

At the salon. Expert techniques offer more variety than home perm products – from root perms for instant lift or waves just at the forehead, to soft bubbles or renaissance style waves on longer hair. They can be made-to-measure for your individual hair type and the look you wish to achieve. Discuss it with your hairdresser – but remember to be honest about products you've used on your hair recently and mention if you've been ill, are taking any drugs, are pregnant or have recently had a baby as this may affect how the perm reacts on your hair.

After your perm. New perms do drop a little after the first week or two, so if it looks a little tight, don't worry. You can revive perms that have flattened overnight by a spray of water and fluffing up with your fingers. As perms grow out, inevitably weight and daily haircare will cause straightening. How often you wish to re-perm depends on the look you wish to achieve. By a different cut, you could lift some of the perm left and you'll discover a new softer style

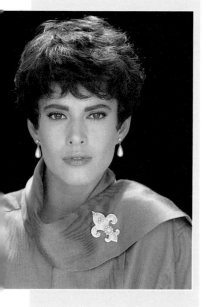

with mousse and scrunching while drying. Or you may wish to just 'lift' the roots where regrowth is straight, leaving the ends wavy. Permed hair does need careful conditioning even though modern ones contain conditioning treatments. Make sure you apply a heavy duty conditioner once a week.

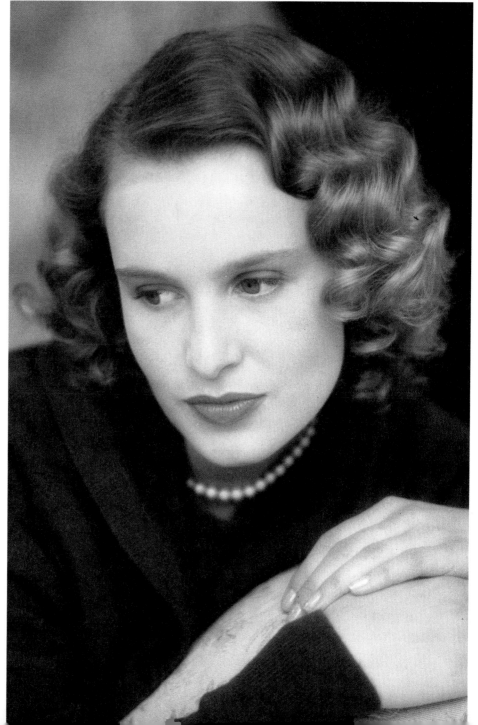

Styling. Like curly hair, permed hair can be made softer by blow drying or kept curly by natural drying with a setting product. Experiment with your new hair.

Relaxing hair

Black afro hair, which is frizzy, can be relaxed and straightened in the same way as hair is made curlier – although it's wise to use a relaxing product made especially for the job. The chemicals reform the hair's structure and then set it straighter with neutraliser when wound on large rollers. If you wish to relax your hair, take the same precautions as for permed hair, remembering to cut and colour afterwards and keep hair in good condition.

Hair colour

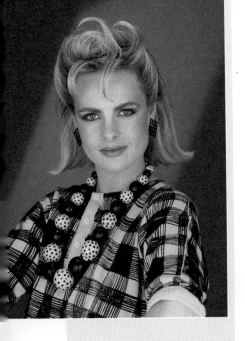

There's nothing like changing your hair colour to brighten up your appearance, add character to your overall look and give you a boost. Although women have changed their hair shade since Roman times (when bright yellow was considered a mark of great beauty), during this century dyed hair has been considered much too bold if it looks coloured – until recently, that is! A few years ago, like cosmetic surgery today, women did not talk about changing their hair colour; it was meant to look natural. Now we're having fun with shades from block black to bleached white blond on younger women and an array of rainbow colours in between. Hair colour has become a fashion accessory and the introduction of the temporary Crazy Colours in the 1970s allowed women simply to wash out one colour and add another each day. Colour, be it temporary, semi-permanent or permanent, is still used like this by many younger people; others use colour to give dull, natural hair colour a lift or add interest through streaks of two or more natural looking shades. Some women use colour to cover grey hair and make them look younger. Armed with the right basic information, anyone can aim for a new shade of hair.

Temporary colour washes out after one shampoo on hair in good condition. Temporary colour simply coats the hair shaft and comes in mousses, gels, wash-in shampoos or spray-on cans.

Semi-permanent colour dyes some of the cuticle, the top layer of the hair, and washes out, fading gradually with each wash over six shampoos. Most also contain conditioners so will make hair look shiny and healthy. Semi-permanents cannot alter the tone of your hair to make it lighter – only permanents can do that. Henna is a semi-permanent.

Permanent colour always requires two products to be mixed together and lasts until you cut off the dyed hair. Permanent colours change the chemical structure of the hair by oxidisation, getting into the hair shaft to dissolve some of your natural colour and replace it with another. You can only change hair back to your natural shade by asking an expert hairdressing technician to replace it with another permanent colour similar to your original one. Permanent colour sometimes fades with damage – for instance, with heated styling products or in the sun.

BEFORE YOU DYE

Whether it be temporary, semi- or permanent colour, make sure that your hair is in good condition and not already coloured. Damaged, dry hair through too much heat, styling, illness or pregnancy, or hair that has already been coloured, will absorb even temporary colour through open damaged cuticles and make it more permanent. If your hair is permed, wait for a few weeks before

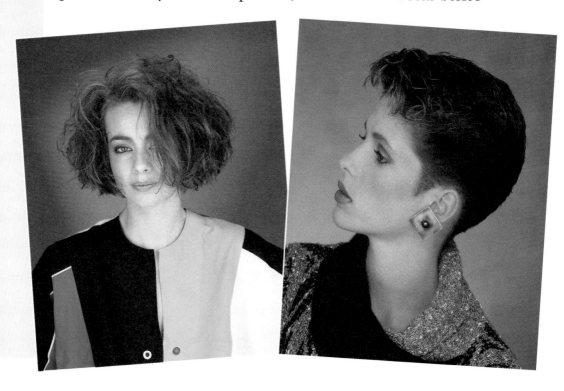

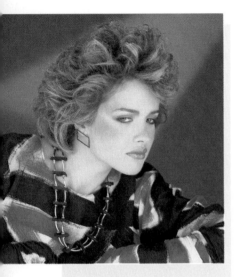

attempting a colour change and use a product which says it can be used on permed hair. Always do a strand test on some hair just above the ear (where it can be covered with other hair but you can still see the shade against your skin tone) at least 24 hours before at-home colouring or ask your hairdresser to do this at a salon, if you're not sure. This will test for allergic reaction as well as allowing you to see what depth of shade suits you. If the strand looks dull and brittle, don't attempt to colour the hair all over.

Choose the shade for you. Temporary and semi-permanent colorants can be washed out quickly and so, if you make a mistake and choose a shade you don't like later, it's not so much of a problem. But if you're considering a permanent colour change it's worth trying on some wigs to see if that shade suits you. Remember your skin tone and eye colour in relation to the new shade and think about your wardrobe, too. Reds can add warmth to pale skins, but avoid them and go for more ashy, icy tones if you've a ruddy complexion. Only very young or very beautiful faces look better with a darker shade. So as you get older, opt for a lighter colour (nature does this for you with grey hair) or one of the same tone (for instance, red tones to mousy hair). The best way to disguise grey hair is with a light vegetable (semi-permanent) dye which will allow your varied natural shades to show through rather than a block colour which looks dense and unnatural. Alternatively dye can be blended in with streaks of different shades between the light and dark tones already in the hair.

At home. The two biggest mistakes people make are using colorants on already damaged hair (a good hairdresser would not allow this, favouring a milder product which adds conditioner at the same time) and not reading and following the instructions properly. It is vital not to colour already-coloured hair – the chemicals used can react with each other and turn out to be a completely different shade altogether (black and blond can make green!). Also, don't leave the colour on for longer than the recommended time. It's not often possible to see what shade you'll be when hair is rinsed and dried while colorant is on. Trust your test strand (do two if you feel the first one isn't the desired depth of colour).

At the hairdresser. Colourists at hairdressers are trained to know what will suit your hair condition, colour and skin tone. Listen to their advice. And if they say don't do it, your hair can't take it – believe them.

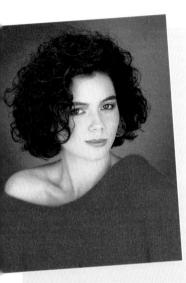

If you want a dramatic look consider several different shades of streaks. Your hair is not the same shade all over (fair-haired people may even find the odd black hair on their heads) and these streaks can look exciting and natural. Or consider just having the ends coloured on a one-length or layered cut. And just one broad streak of colour looks dramatic on a shiny geometric cut.

If you don't want roots showing any permanent colour will require root retouching after a while. Shorter cuts show up a different root colour quicker than long hair. Highlights don't show them up so quickly; nor does just a shade darker or lighter than

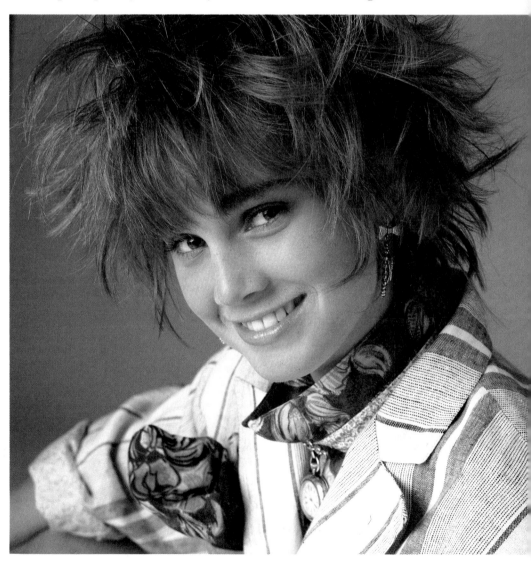

your natural one. Average root retouching time for highlighted hair is six weeks, but it's more likely to be three or less for all-over colour which is a complete change from your normal one. Consider this when you decide to dye. Ask a hairdresser for costs to root retouch and how often and long it's likely to take each time before you invest.

Going blond. It's the most popular shade of all. Anyone from redhead to mousy, brown to fair can achieve lighter hair which looks natural, and highlights are the most popular option. Dark hair can look dramatically different with blond streaks but this won't suit

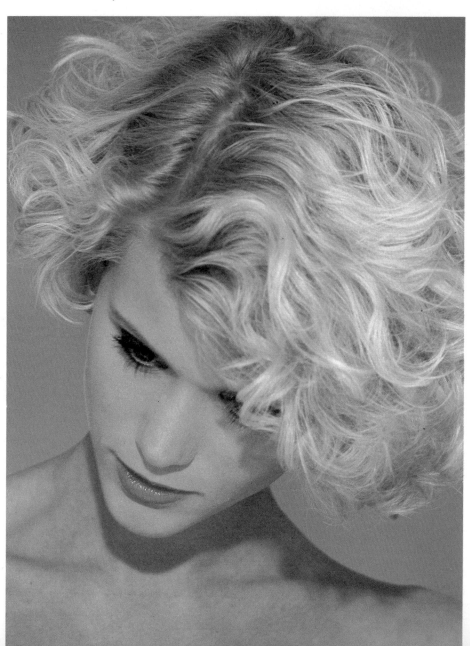

everyone. And grey hair can look brighter and younger if it takes on a honey tone. Remember that the sun lightens hair naturally and so it's worth having hair lightened *after* a holiday when it helps to keep the sunkissed look for longer.

A change of style

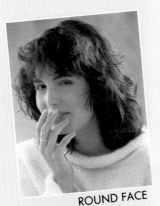

ROUND FACE

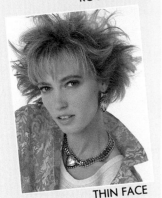

THIN FACE

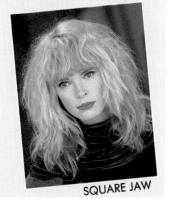

SQUARE JAW

The cut. Your hair will naturally suit some styles (for instance, thin straight hair suits an easy-to-keep chin-length bob; wavy hair can be shown off with a graduated layered style). Other looks may need more styling each time you wash your hair. Firstly, decide how long you can spend styling your hair at each shampoo; do you need to wash your hair frequently because you play a lot of sport? Do you need an uncrushable style because you have to wear a hat or cap for work? The answer may be a perm, straightening or colour to go with your new cut.

Now you have to decide what shape of cut will suit you. For instance, large voluminous hair will make smaller, rounder figures look even rounder, while a close crop will give a pinhead effect – this shape needs a mid-length hair style. Tall, thin people can get away with a wider variety of styles but can look too much like a beanpole with a short crop. Then there's your face shape: round faces look better with graduated bouncy styles with height on top to thin the overall outline. Long, thin faces need horizontal lines like a fringe or some width above ear level to balance them. Square faces with pronounced jawlines should choose a style that brings hair on to the face and below the chin, softening those angular lines; height on top helps, too. Spectacle-wearers have a double problem; they'll need to choose their specs and hairstyle to suit their face shape and go with each other; the best plan is to make a feature of glasses by taking hair away from them.

Now you're ready to discuss a new style with your hairdresser. Go into the salon dressed in your usual style of clothes and make-up, to give the hairdresser some idea of how you normally look. Let him know if you'd be nervous about a dramatic change or if there's one of your features that you'd like to disguise (a large nose, wide cheekbones and so on). A picture from a magazine often helps communication and, although (as said before) your hairdresser may not be able to achieve this *exactly*, it will give him some idea of the style that you're after.

The large picture shows long, thick hair with some natural wave. Use mousse, gel, straightening tongs and hair accessories such as bands and clips to achieve the styles shown in the smaller pictures.

The styling. The hairdresser who cuts your hair is also the best person to ask about styling and changing the style of that particular cut. It may even be worthwhile taking along an accessory (such as a comb or hat) that you like to wear and asking how you can adapt your hairstyle to it. There are many, many products on the market to help you achieve a different look with your hair. Apart from mousses, gels and styling sprays to give volume, smoothness and wave and keep it there, discover the options given by heated appliances such as crimpers, straighteners, diffusers (for scrunch

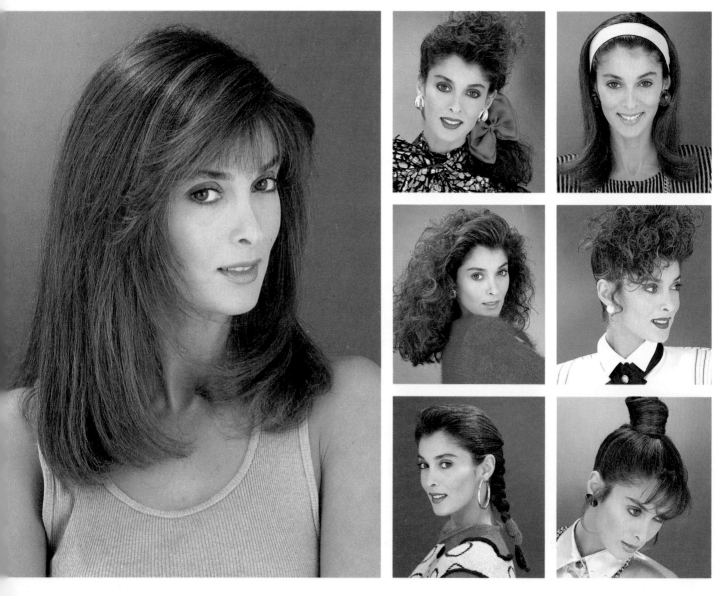

The large picture shows fine straight hair in a bob type cut. The smaller pictures illustrate how versatile this style can be using imagination and hair products available at any large chemist.

drying or more natural curls), heated rollers, curling tongs or brushes.

The secret of success is to experiment. Don't immediately go and buy all these products, but instead, with advice on the possibilities suitable for your hair from your hairdresser, borrow one from a friend for the evening and make full use of it. Then you'll find out if the investment is worthwhile. Try, for instance, twisting strands of long hair before rolling them round a heated roller or curling tongs or gelling smooth short hair and then creating ripples with

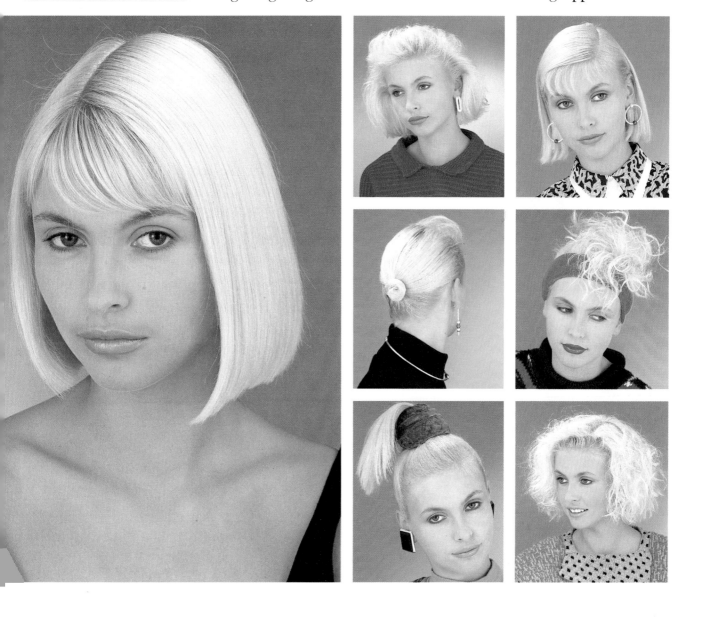

the side of your hand. Use mousse on damp hair with a diffuser attachment to your hairdryer to scrunch medium length, layered hair and make it look wild and fluffy. Try a smaller rounded brush with your dryer to curl underneath hair to give more height to top hair. Or make curls forwards and sideways, instead of backwards, with a curling wand to achieve a different hairline around the face. But remember that heated styling aids and, to some extent, mousses and gels (find the ones with added conditioners) can dry out and damage fine, permed or colour-treated hair, so try not to use them at every wash; and when you do use heat and styling products to achieve your look, make sure you condition well beforehand to help protect hair.

Some style ideas

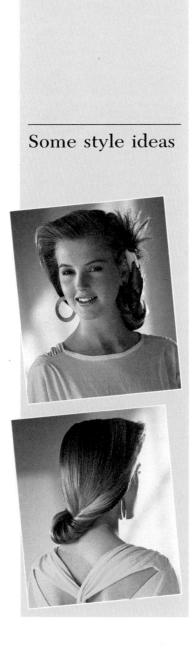

- Make long hair look short. Gather ends and twist into a rope. Pin to back of head leaving enough loose to frizz into spikes on top of your crown.
- Don't use elastic bands to tie back long hair; they apply too much pressure and can break hairs. Instead, use specially made covered bands, ribbons, scarves or 'butterfly' clips.
- Get instant fullness by styling damp hair into narrow woven plaits over your head. Leave overnight to dry, then brush out for a wild look. This style is great for giving extra body to fine hair.
- A tip from Grandma – give overnight wave by rag curling. Cut old sheets into strips and roll damp hair round them. Tie two ends close to your head when fully wound. Wait until hair is dry before taking out strips and brushing.
- Gentle waves? Try pin curling by winding small sections of damp hair into loose curls round your finger. Fasten with a grip and leave to dry – you can even sleep as they set.
- You don't have to wet hair to set it with rollers but, if it's dry, a spray of water reactivates setting lotions, gels or mousse and helps the curls to stay.
- Prevent rollered hair from going flat at the roots during the day by pulling strands at right angles away from your scalp before winding.
- Wrap tissue or perming paper round tips of hair when using heated rollers to prevent the drier ends being directly applied to heat.
- Long hair can be fun with a very simple accessory such as a stretchy hairband which can be worn in different ways. Use it as an Alice band to keep hair off face. Use it to tie hair in a pretty side ponytail. Wear it as a sweatband and backcomb fringe above it to complete the style.

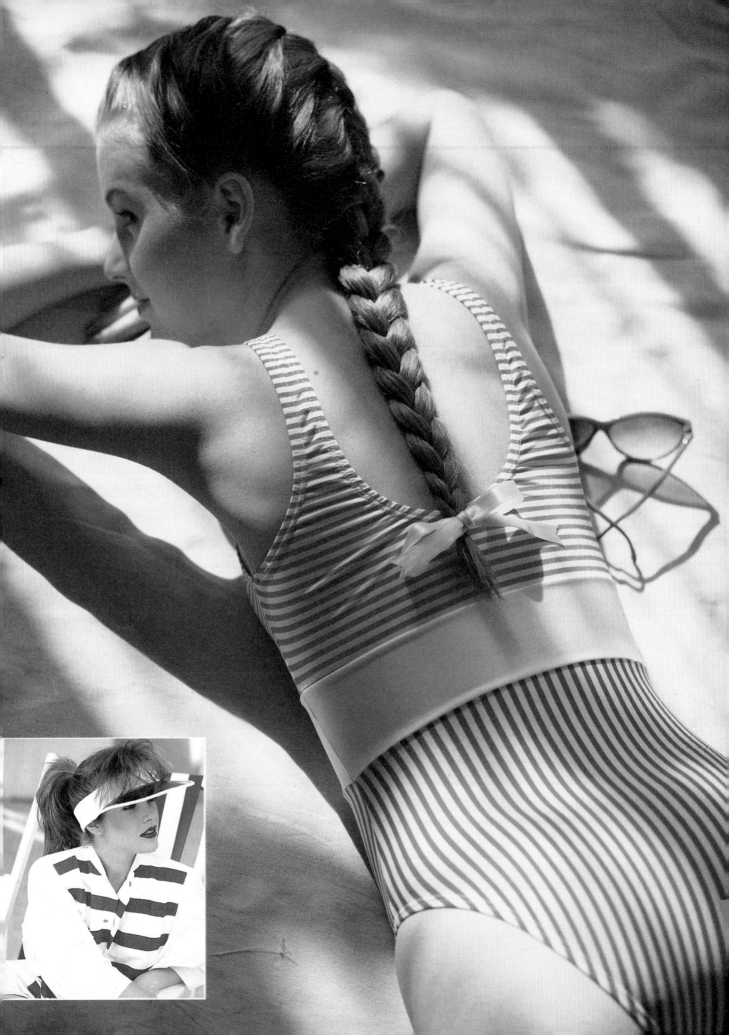

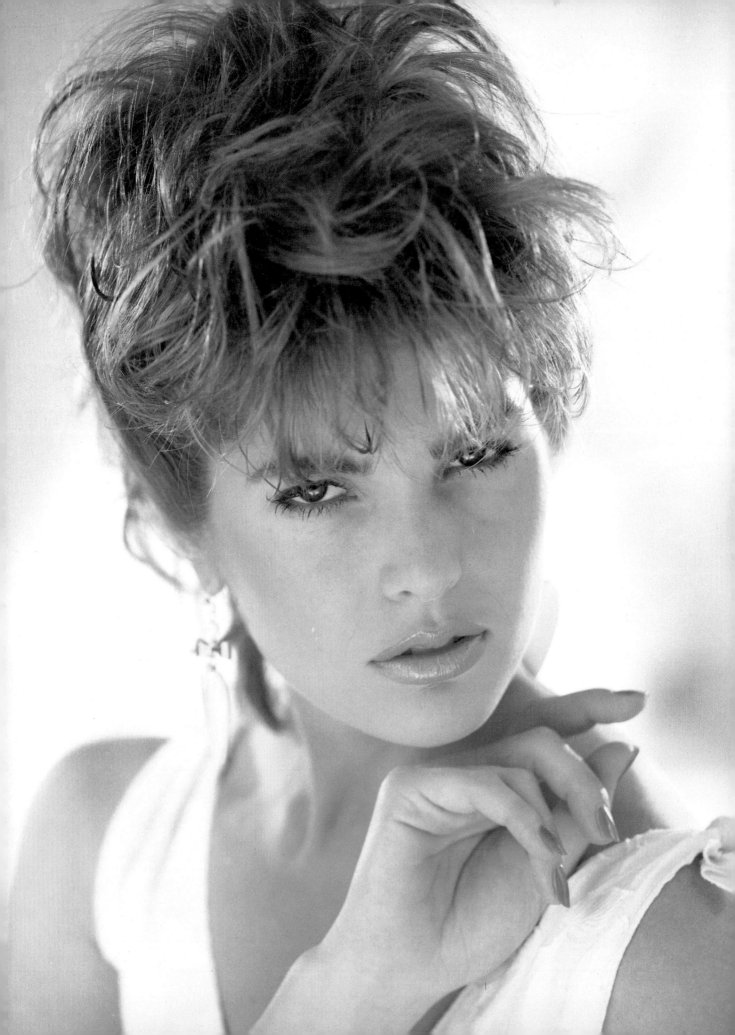

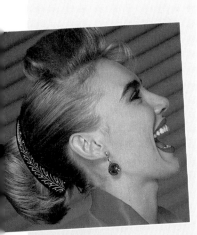

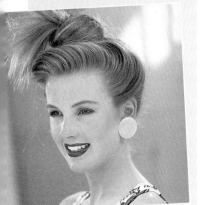

Unusual hair accessories can make your style look different. Paint an old-fashioned clothes' peg bright yellow or red, tie hair back with segments of bright or sparkly tights or use jewellery for glamour.

For shorter hair which is growing out of a perm or colour or is just greasy, tie a pretty scarf round your head and pull a few wisps through on to the face for softness. Match scarf colour to your make-up or outfit.

For hair growing out of a perm, comb straight back using gel to help smooth it, then tie hair with a big coloured bow or bunch of ribbons to get an impression of length.

For medium-length hair which you're trying to grow, hide uneven layers by making two side twists. Simply take hair in your hands at either side of the face and twist into a small rope, pinning it behind the twist so pins don't show. When you let this style loose, it will be curly. Add more volume with a handful of mousse.

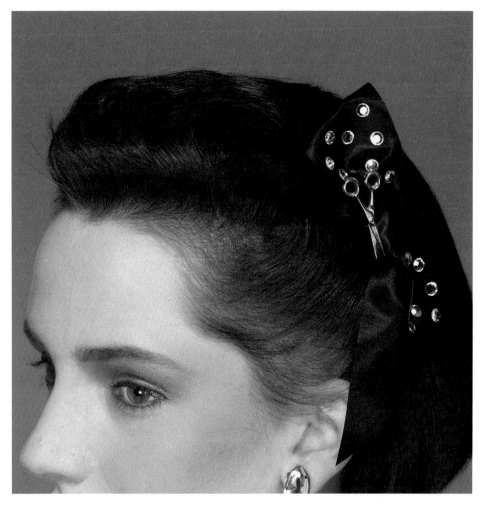

False hair

False pieces and wigs can look natural to cover hair or scalp
problems or to achieve a different look. Or they can be deliberately
false for the pure fun of it. Natural-looking hairpieces and wigs look
best when they're in a similar colour to your own hair and so match
the skintone and eye colouring which suit your normal hair. Obvious
false pieces can be of any colour from glittering gold to bleached
blond or pink. The best way to attach a false piece that you wish to
look like your hair is to incorporate it into your own. Make the
hairpiece a ponytail, wrapping your own hair round the band before
securing it with a grip. Now you can create a bun or top knot, if you
wish. Half-head false pieces are also available for making hair look
thicker – a trick used by celebrities. Attach them at the back just
below your crown and simply brush natural hair over them. Try
weaving false pieces into your own hairstyle, too – imagine a black
plait with a blue strand running through it, or a wild style with locks
of red running through blond hair.

Wigs should be chosen extra carefully if they're meant to look
natural. Whether they're made of real or synthetic hair, you can
style them in various ways, just like your own head of hair. Wigs
look more realistic if hair comes forwards over the face, especially at
the forehead, so that you can't see a definite hairline, which on your
natural hair is not as uniform as on a manufactured wig.

The male of the species

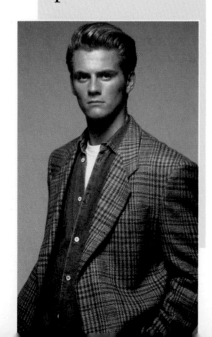

As men's hair is no different in texture and type from women's, the
same rules apply to keeping it in good condition. The only
difference that men should be aware of is that thinning, receding
and balding hair should not be over-processed with chemicals such
as colour and perms. Too many of these processes can weaken hair
at the roots even further. An expert perm a little away from the
roots can make thinning hair look thicker. And vegetable dye, which
doesn't alter the hair chemically, can disguise grey hair but fades
gradually and needs re-application every six weeks or so.

Short hair shows grease and a flaking scalp quickly, so regular
washing and brushing are a must for a healthy-looking head. A good
hairstyle will help change and flatter face shape, emphasising nice
features and playing down bad ones. Any hairdresser worth knowing

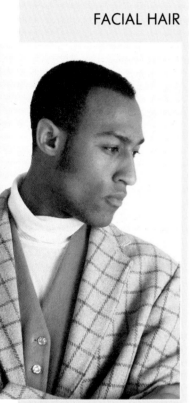

should be able to advise about how gels and setting aids can give a new style to a basic cut.

FACIAL HAIR

Men who decide to wear a beard and/or moustache must make sure it looks good by keeping it clean and well groomed. A beard needs to be washed in shampoo every day (the skin underneath needs cleaning and beards do tend to collect food and debris!). It needs trimming at least every six weeks to stay in shape, and longer beards should be brushed regularly. Special razors are available to keep the 'designer stubble' look in trim for those who like this style.

Long sideboards aren't fashionable now. They can be kept in trim with a razor. Sore skin can be eased with a warm soapy soak just before shaving to soften hair and make it easier to cut; follow with a soothing aftershave balm to calm and cool. Astringent aftershave lotions can irritate skin made more sensitive by being scraped.

It is worth plucking heavy eyebrows; especially if they meet in the middle to give a permanent frown. Soak the area with a warm flannel for a few minutes. Then, using flat-ended tweezers, grip each hair individually near the base and pull it sharply in the direction it is going. Afterwards, cool with a splash of cold water. Redness takes a few hours to go initially but hairs will get less resilient as you re-pluck. Trim unsightly nasal and ear hair with a fine but blunt-ended pair of cosmetic scissors.

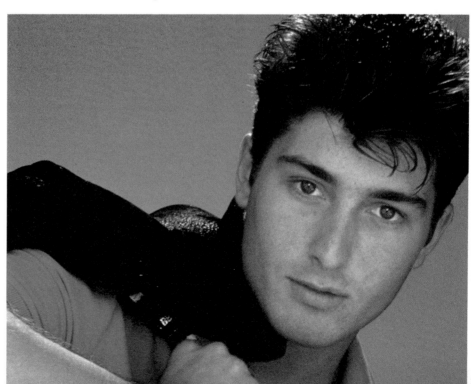

CHAPTER 4

The Wonderful World of Colour

For centuries human beings have adorned their bodies and painted their faces with colour. The reasons why are almost as varied as the looks that resulted. Originally, males probably used colour for camouflage while hunting; later to show tribal identification, for status, in warfare and for religious or magical ceremony.

Throughout the centuries, painting skin has also been used to create and enhance beauty. The Ancient Egyptians found that pigments protected their skins from the sun, particularly around the eyes. These colours around the eyes also made them look brighter and more beautiful and so eye painting became a popular cosmetic pursuit. We still find painted eyes beautiful but some past beauty looks are less easy to understand. Who would wish to copy the red-stained teeth of Hindu women or black-stained teeth of the Japanese in a modern world? Yet in some countries still, the tracing of veins in blue dye, elaborate tattooing over forehead, nose and cheeks, henna-stained red feet and hands, black faces painted chalky white, cheeks scarred with lines at birth or saucer-size bottom lips are considered smart and attractive.

It's only during this century that men in the Western world have lost interest in facial decoration. In earlier eras powdered wigs and faces, along with beauty spots, rouged lips and cheeks, indicated a chap at the height of fashion. Nowadays women have certainly overtaken them. Never before has there been such a choice of products with which to camouflage and paint the face. In the late 1930s Max Factor brought the panstick off the stage and made it available to ordinary women. More lipstick shades than the conventional red became easily available. Browns, mauves and turquoises were added to the conventional blue and green eyeshadows. Then, in the 1960s, Mary Quant and Biba burst on to the market with crayons to paint your face and a whole assortment of new nail and lip shades (such as silver, green and black) which matched your clothes and changed with the season. Rouge, which had become unfashionable a decade or more before, was transformed into blusher or shaders and introduced to the mass market to shade and shape the face.

We haven't looked back since. Make-up has survived (along with the bra) the women's liberation movement of the seventies and is used by feminists in the eighties. Unlike earlier years, when certain classes did or didn't wear make-up according to convention, these liberated days provide choice. There are no social rules for wearing

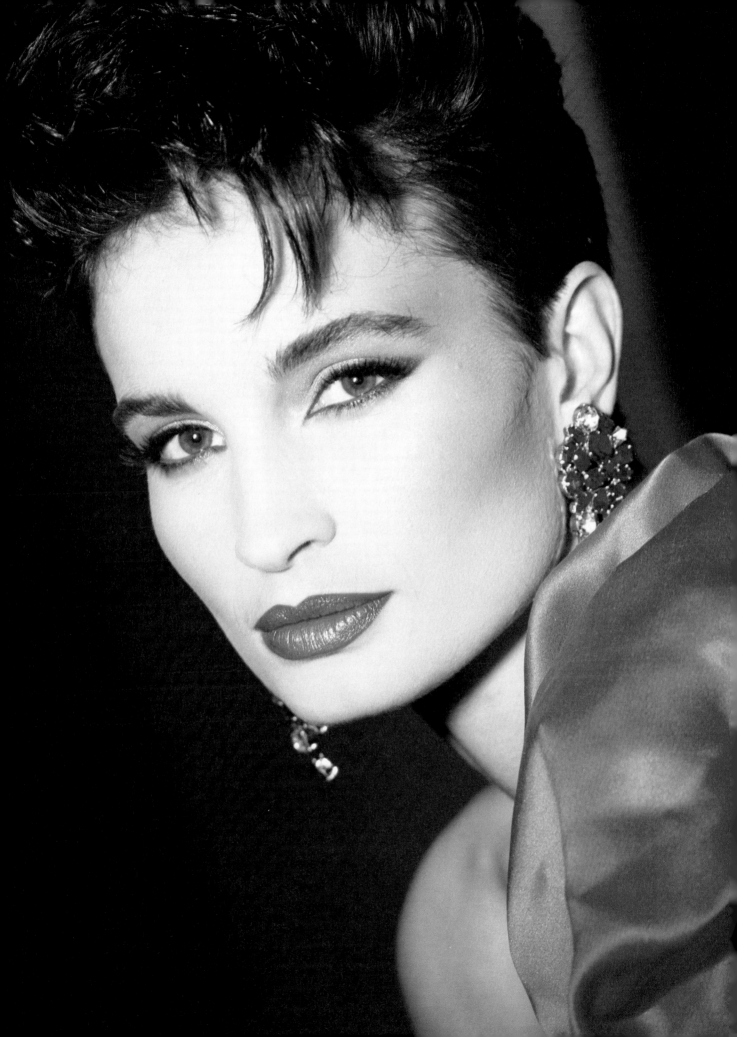

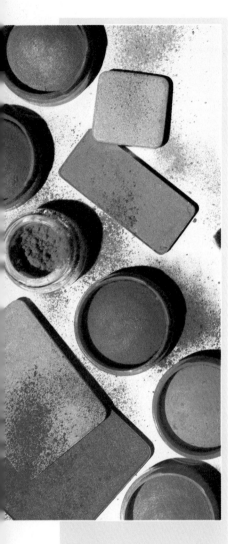

or not wearing make-up. Those women who don't want to are not considered unconventional, as they may once have been. Those who do or do some of the time can play it up, punk style, without causing too much of a rumpus or keep it subtle in an attempt to flatter their features and sometimes to make them look younger.

Make-up without the rules is special and fun to those who wear it, and like any pleasurable pursuit, only becomes sinister when the doer can't do without it. Beauty editors are often accused of suggesting that women 'need' make-up and are somehow reduced without it. This stems from those few unfortunate women who lack self-esteem and come to rely on face painting as a mask, afraid to be seen in their natural state – be it by the milkman, their family or friends. But cosmetic junkies are few and far between and it's possible these women would have leant on another, probably more dangerous, crutch if make-up hadn't been at hand.

In some cases make-up can be psychologically beneficial. Red Cross beauticians not only go into hospitals to cheer up patients by making them look and feel more attractive but also give advice on disguising scars, birthmarks or other facial disfigurements. They have proved that these services help the ill to recover quicker from operations and lift depression due to feelings of unattractiveness. But for most of us make-up, like fashion, is something you decide to use to flatter or make you more fashionable. No one, and certainly not society, is demanding that you must wear it.

Most women enjoy adorning themselves with some kind of colour. It makes them feel more attractive or allows them to have fun playing roles – the sophisticated woman, the country girl, the extrovert, the fashion setter, the siren. Make-up can be used to make us look younger, less tired or as a disguise for bad skin. It can emphasise a facial feature that we're proud of while distracting attention from one we're not. All you need is your painting equipment and a good canvas (the best skin possible) to let loose your artistic talents.

Your bag of tricks and the games they can play

Apart from the colours you apply to your face, choosing what to put them on with can make the difference between a botch job or a work of art. Of course, your own expertise will come into how attractive or stunning the overall look is but by selecting the right tools of the trade, you're giving yourself a head start.

FACE AND NECK

A mini-sponge. Foundation, whether it be liquid or solid, is best applied with a damp sponge. This will help the foundation to go on smoothly and evenly and make sure it reaches into corners (such as the sides of your nose). A make-up sponge can either be a mini natural sponge found in larger department stores or health shops or a synthetic one (sometimes sold with the base foundation product). The most important point is that the texture should be fine (without large holes in it). Always rinse them out before use, squeezing through with tepid, clear water to remove dirt or preservatives and soften them up. Then squeeze until just damp and put liquid foundation into the palm of a clean hand, dabbing the sponge into it. With solid, palette type foundations, dab the damp sponge on to them before stroking and blending into the face.

A fine, short-haired brush. Used artfully, it can be loaded with concealer or a paler foundation for covering up spots and blemishes, deeper wrinkles and red veins. Just dab on to the area to be covered and blend the edges into the skin.

A velvety compact puff or a huge soft brush. Dipped into soft or drawn over solid powder, tapped to remove excess and then stroked over foundation, it will help set it and give a good base for further colour.

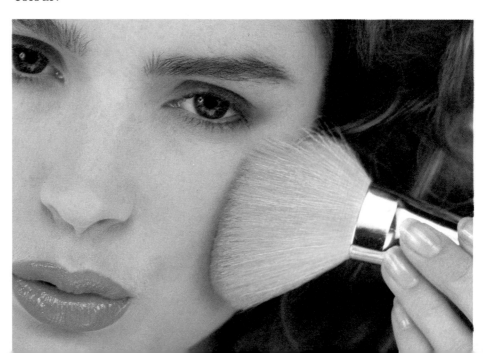

A *rounded, soft, large brush* for applying blusher and shading the face. It allows good contour power without harsh lines. Use sweeping strokes from the centre of face outwards. Cream blushers should be dotted along cheekbones, then patted and blended with pads of fingertips.

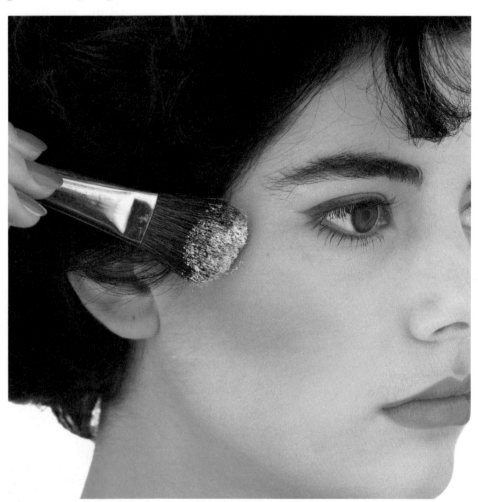

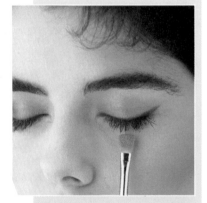

EYES

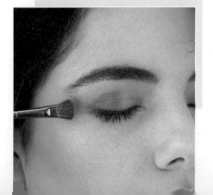

Sponge-tip applicators or smaller tufted eyeshadow brushes should be tested for softness on the inside wrist before buying. Often eyeshadows come with applicators but with many of the less expensive brands they are too rough. The eye area is one of the most delicate, and harsh applicators or bristles will irritate the skin here. If you use large eye-shading pencils for shadow, you'll also

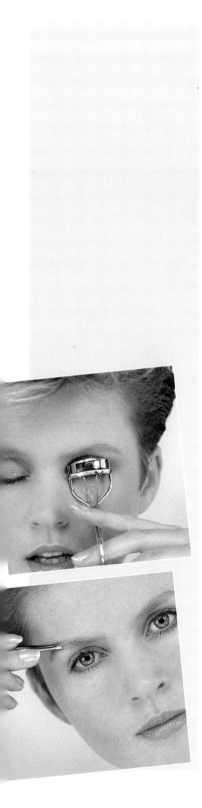

need a large cosmetic sharpener for greater accuracy. Applicators are good for applying block colour over lid or under brow. Brushes can do this, too, and are more adept at blending two shades together where they meet. Stroke them across powder shadows and tap lightly to remove excess. To apply shadow use short, soft strokes (with cream or powder shadows) across lid from inside to out. Remember to wipe several times across a tissue before using the same brush for another powder shade. Applicators and brushes used for cream shadows are best used just for the same shade each time as colour tends to cling, although you can wash them (see below).

A *fine eyeliner brush*, used instead of a pencil, gives precise application of liquid eyeliner as close to lashes as possible. Dry on a tissue and stroke over the line again to soften the look. Alternatively, place dots of eyeliner between lashes with the pointed tip of the brush and blend together with the dry brush for a defining rather than a lined look.

Eyelash and brow comb. This double-sided comb has a mini rigid comb on one side to separate lashes clogged with thickly applied or too liquid mascara. The mini brush on the other side straightens and grooms eyebrow hairs. Use the brush upwards at the centre of your brow, slanting it sideways as you go out towards the outer eyebrow.

Eyelash curlers look like instruments of Chinese torture but in fact are painless, instant lash crimpers. They act like non-cutting scissors as you clamp top lashes between the blades for a count of 10, either before or – if lashes are hard to curl – after, applying mascara. They will crease eyelash ends upwards making them look longer and more visible. They are available at large chemists and you can replace the rubber clamps when they wear down. Wash with warm soapy water or surgical spirit (but make sure this dries completely before using again).

Tweezers. Those with wedge ends are less dangerous and easier for plucking eyebrow hairs. Whether you decide that your eyebrows need thinning or not, stray hairs too near the lid crease, between the brows or outside the eye corner can hinder the effect of a beautiful eye make-up. Hairs should be plucked in the direction of hair growth in good light (daylight is best) and preferably after soaking the area with a warm flannel to help open pores. Never overpluck these beauty assets: thicker eyebrows help to define and emphasise eye shape. Dab with toner or cold water to help constrict pores again.

LIPS

A *short tufted wedge-shaped brush* is dual purpose. Use the thin wedge end to outline lips just by wiping the brush over lipstick and then contouring a lipline (if you use lip pencils you will need a sharpener instead). The fine flat part adds colour inside the line. Alternatively use a pointed (eyeliner) brush for lining and a small rounded one for filling in.

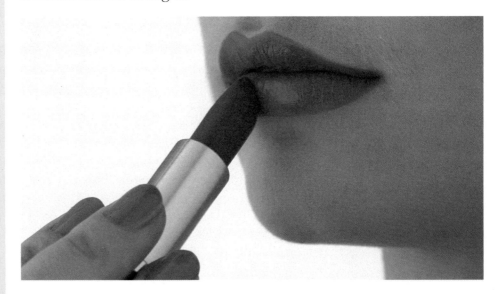

TAKE-OFF

One of the most important aspects of make-up is to give yourself the ideal base to work on and this means taking off old or surplus make-up effectively before applying new (see Chapter 2 for cleansing information). Cotton wool is not an ideal tool for taking off cleanser, as the tiny filaments can fall into your eyes and irritate them. Tissues don't absorb enough to remove *heavy* make-up and can disintegrate. The best take-off tool is the relatively new cotton wool pads, made especially for the purpose and packed closely with absorbent cotton so that they don't fluff off with use. Dampening them slightly with warm water helps the whole process, too.

CLEANING YOUR TOOLS

Like any good artist, you need to keep your equipment in pristine condition for it to give you maximum wear and effectiveness. A good make-up bag should be waterproof inside so spills and leaks can be easily wiped away. Just turn the bag inside out and wipe over with warm, soapy water. Do this regularly. At the same time take the opportunity to clean messy make-up containers and applicator handles. Brushes should be wiped clean against a tissue dampened with carbon tetrachloride (the dry cleaning solution) once a week if you wear make-up every day. You can wash them in warm soapy water but this removes oil from natural hair, and some glues which hold the bristles to the base dissolve in water – so be warned! After cleaning, work bristles into the shape of the brush and allow them to dry off naturally. Never scrub them or allow them to stand head down so the brush loses its shape. Clean sponge tools in warm water with a dash of washing-up liquid, squeezing the sponge through to remove any pigment and oil left in it. Rinse thoroughly and allow to dry naturally. Heat will harden synthetic tools and roughen natural hair ones.

Cosmetics: the options

Foundations are oil-in-water or water-in-oil mixtures containing varying degrees of pigment to give your skin an even tone throughout and a base on which to apply other colours. Choose your foundation by finding the same skintone as your face on your inside or outside wrist. Now establish whether your skintone is basically pink (ruddy, tendency to high colour), yellow (pale, tendency to ghostly) or, with black skin, it may also be blue/grey based. Select a shade of foundation in your group (pink, yellow or blue-based) as near to your own skintone as possible, remembering to reassess the shade after a sunshine holiday, when you have a fading tan or after a long dull winter when skin is extra pale. Try the foundation on your wrist where skin matches face colour and look at the effect in daylight before deciding whether to buy. It's also worth leaving it on for some hours to discover whether it sinks in well or how long the pigment lasts. Although your wrist skin is not often precisely the same as your face in its acid/alkali balance, this will give you some idea of how the product performs.

Tinted moisturisers aren't really foundations, as the aim is to moisturise rather than colour. They give just a hint of pigment and so this need not match your skintone too precisely. A deep tan moisturiser can make your skin look slightly sun-tanned with your natural colour showing through. Tinted moisturisers can be used instead of an ordinary moisturiser during the day if you don't want skin cover or disguise. Some have the added advantage of containing sunscreen.

Light foundations contain more pigment, and although their aim is to even up skintone, they won't help disguise obvious marks. The most liquid of the foundation group, they sink into the skin while helping to even up skintone and give a good luminous glow.

Thicker foundations are creamier and sometimes solid, in a palette type container. They're ideal for dry skins as they don't sink in so easily but help to protect and seal skin. Their heavy coverage will help to disguise blemishes or dark under-eye circles and they can make skin look extra glamorous for evenings and special occasions.

Mauve, green and white bases tone down and even out complexion problems. Mauve and green bases tone down a skin that tends to redden or has broken veins – foundation goes on top. White bases give extra cover and add a luminous glow to skintone – either apply before foundation or mix with it.

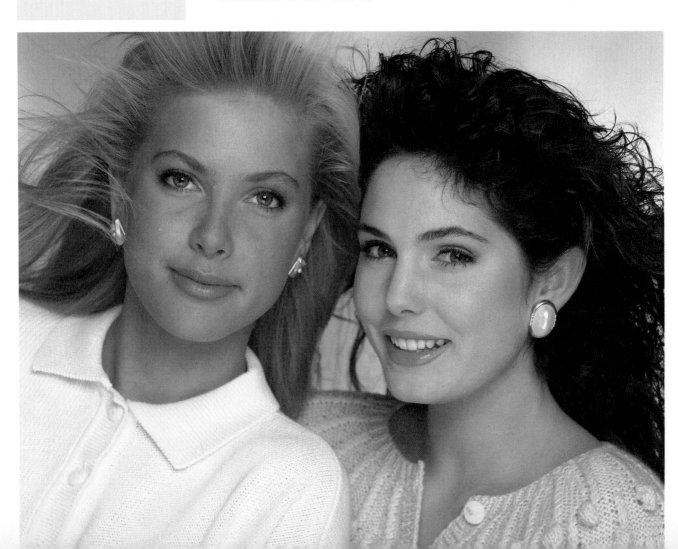

Concealers, used artfully, can disguise spots, birthmarks, scars and, to some extent, deeper wrinkles. Choosing the colour is all-important; aim for one shade lighter than your skintone, use a matt covering foundation in a shade lighter than your usual foundation if you can't find the right shade. Apply with the applicator provided, clean fingertips or a thin brush (especially for wrinkles where the aim is to lighten the dark, indented groove). Blend by patting into the skin at the edges of the blemish and cover with foundation. You may need to touch up again, over foundation.

Powders 'set' foundation and rid your face of shine, giving it a matt look. Powders should never be rubbed on; instead, dust with short, soft strokes so as not to disturb foundation. Make sure you don't put on too much powder by tapping the puff or brush before applying. Colour choice can be translucent which, as the name suggests, allows your foundation shade to show through, or matching foundation and chosen in the same way.

Brushing and shading. Contouring your face with blushers can disguise features you want to hide (a long nose, a weak chin) and bring out ones that you're proud of (wide cheekbones, a pretty forehead). Cream blushers are less popular these days and should be applied before powder. Powder blushers come in almost every shade of red, pink, brown and orange under the sun. Basically, the darker the shade the more they'll make shadows (lighter ones should be reserved for highlighting areas you want to stand out – for instance, the top of the cheekbones, centre of forehead). Contour just under cheekbones from mid under eye, where cheekbone starts, to temple for definition. Wide foreheads can be concealed and flattered with darker blushers at each temple. Use a tawny shade under the tip of a long nose or down the sides of a wide one to lessen the look. Under a pointed chin or along a loose jawline the same shade will make the chin look softer, the jaw stronger. These disguises will be too visible for everyday or daylight make-ups. They are best used, after a lot of practice with blending to get the most natural-looking effect, for evening or electric light.

EYES

Cream eyeshadows have also lost popularity in recent years as they're not so versatile, but if you use them they should go on before powder and be retouched afterwards. Eye make-up very much depends on the individual shape but there are a few tricks which flatter all eyes. Taking three shadows: a light, medium and dark in contrasting or matching colours, apply the medium one over your eyelid to the crease. Then apply the lighter one at the brow – above the crease and below your eyebrow. The darker shade is then softly stroked (not too heavily) along the crease from mid-lid out to flick up at the end towards the brow. Use a clean brush to blend these shadows where they meet. The darker shade can also be used with a fine brush and water as an eyeliner round the outside corner lashline. A variation on this basic theme for wide-spaced eyes is to apply the darker shadow at the inner lid area blending into the nose to 'pull' the eyes together. Alternatively, the lighter shade can add extra emphasis to lids and under the eye with one dot on the centre lid and lots of small ones between lower lashes.

A few tips:

- Very few people suit the original pale blue or green shadows. Instead match eye colours to your clothes, jewellery, hair or even nail shades.
- Matt shades blend together better. Save the sparkly or pearly shadows for one all-over eye colour.
- Safest eye colours for those who aren't so good at matching are skintone shades: beiges, peaches, pale dusky pinks, browns, tans. Alternatively, look at the flecks in your iris (instead of the whole colour) and try to match these.
- Experiment; you can always wipe it off. Put too much on and then tone it down by brushing over with a clean brush. When you go out, wear too little rather than too much in daylight and too much rather than too little at night or in electric light.
- Mascara can look overdone on long lashes. Try non-build-up ones (without filaments) or leave lower lashes mascara free, if they're dark.

LIPS

Fashions come and go in lipshades more than anywhere else. But it's up to you to decide whether you want your mouth or your eyes to be the main focus of your face and then play up one or the other. If you feel your eyes are your best feature practise with lots of colour and extra definition. And if you're not proud of your lip or nose shape, it's wise to aim for a more subtle lip shade so this area is less noticeable. Deeper colours can even up an irregular lip line or make lips look larger or smaller.

Always take foundation over lips and powder before applying lip colour. Then, using a pencil or fine brush, paint in the line – around your regular line if you're happy with it, just inside a larger lip line to make it smaller or just outside to make it larger (you can correct an uneven bow or thinner bottom lip by applying this principle to the relevant area, too). Now fill in the lip colour. For extra staying power, blot with a tissue and reapply (see the step-by-step pictures). For sparkle, add a touch of highlighter along the centre of the lower lip or at the bow of the upper lip to make them look prettier and poutier!

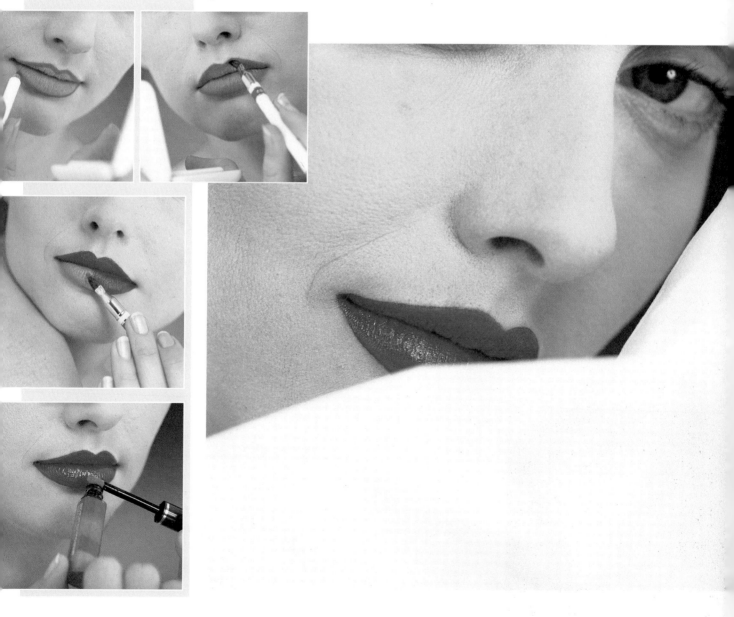

Not the classic pale face?

Black skins

These are lucky in that they have a better barrier function and so retain moisture more efficiently than paler ones. This is because there's a thicker top layer, which could explain why darker skins usually seem to age more slowly. But in cold weather, dryness will show up as a dusty grey tone, so stick to cream cleansers and cleansing bars instead of soaps and try using a light moisturising base underneath your make-up.

Base. There are over 30 shades of darker-than-white skins (and only six white shades), so finding the right foundation can be a trial. Also, uneven pigmentation can mean matching is even more difficult. It's always best to choose from a range specially for black skins as those made for paler skins contain too much white and pink and can make you look 'ghostly'. To select the right shade, match a foundation to the palest area, using a cover stick to hide blemishes beforehand. If you have an oily skin you can set your make-up with a powder over foundation. A translucent one is best if you can't find your exact skin shade.

Eyes. Steer clear of sparkly pearl and very pale colours. Matt colours in deep pigments are much better as skin has its own natural shine. Emphasise eyes with a fine line of liquid liner.

Cheeks. Russet blushers are best for cheekbones. Avoid ones with shimmer in them.

Lips. Line lips for extra definition with a lip pencil a shade darker than your lipstick. Steer clear of mauve shades which aren't so flattering. Try coral, peach, russet and rich brown lip colours instead.

Dusky olive skin tones

Characteristic of Mediterranean and Asian origins, these vary in tone as much as black skins. They range from pale yellow to deeper olive tones, and white skins may take on these shades when tanned.

Base. Skin can look sallow if you choose the wrong base, and if you're not careful you can even look orange! A tinted day cream should be enough to give a healthy glow, but avoid anything with pink tones in it. Use a tinted powder to set this base.

Eyes. Avoid reds, golden yellows and bright blues. Red and yellow will highlight yellow skin tones while blues are too garish.

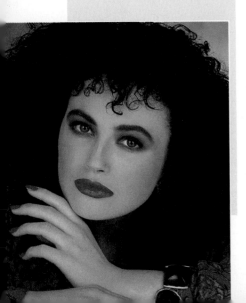

Try instead cool shades such as mauve or moss green on eyelids. The traditional black kohl looks lovely and highlights eyes – smudge it as liner for a softer effect.

Cheeks. A deep rosy/beige blusher will add warmth.

Lips. Shimmery shades look great, or go for reds, browns and plums.

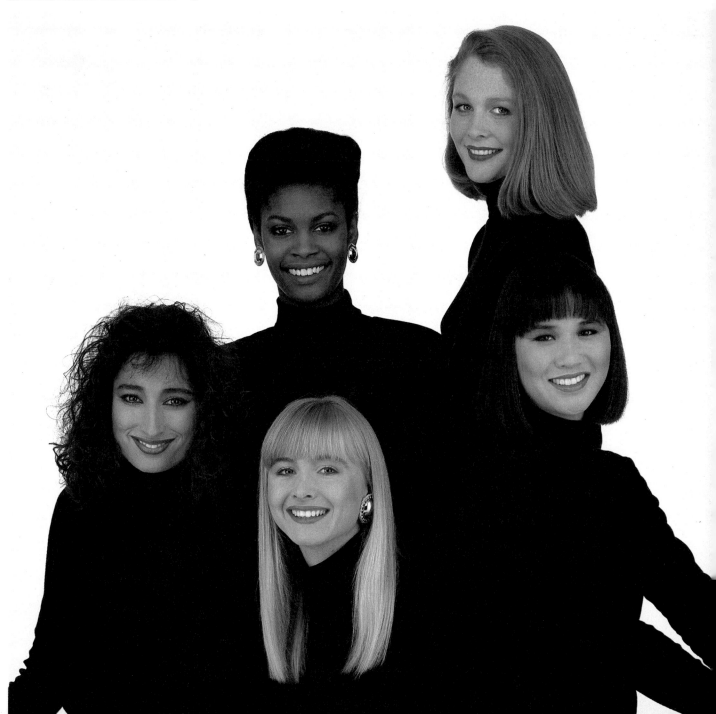

Very pale skin

Combined with white blond hair this can leave you looking washed out, while too much make-up can give the look of a doll. The Nordic complexion is pale with pink and blue skin tones and often very rosy cheeks. Skin is sensitive to both heat and light, so in summer go for a high protection sunscreen. As this skin tends to show up blemishes easily, foundation is important. A green base underneath helps disguise red blotches and blue veins. Cover with a pale ivory foundation or a lightly tinted moisturiser. A white or translucent powder will remove shine. To give skin colour in summer, dust on a tinted glowing powder.

Eyebrows. Darken with brown or grey eyebrow pencil.

Eyes. Anything goes with blondes, but you shouldn't wear too much green and blue to emphasise blue eyes as they can look too hard. Shimmering eye colours in grey, pink and lilac look cool and

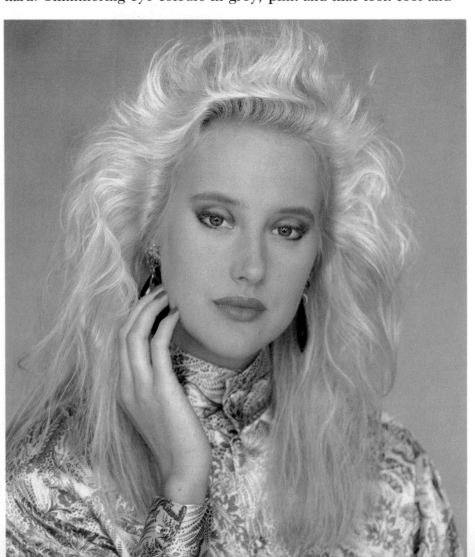

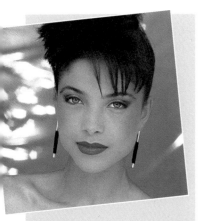

pretty; while browns, beiges and golds add warmth to your face. Darken lashes with grey, brown or navy mascara and, to emphasise eyes, smudge brown kohl pencil beneath lower lashes.

Cheeks. Pale pinks and apricots are the colours to choose but keep blusher to a minimum to avoid looking flushed.

Lips. Opt for pale pinks or coral shades. Steer clear of bright reds or deep brown and plum colours – they look too heavy on pale skins.

Oriental skins

These usually have lovely, even pigmentation and are often smooth and so a heavy make-up base shouldn't be necessary. Wide cheekbones also mean that oriental-shaped faces are lucky in that they don't tend to wrinkle so easily with age.

Base. Skin usually has a blue or yellow tone in it (hold your hand against a stark white wall to see which yours is, then you can match your foundation to it). Stick to pale shades, opting for olive and ivory rather than pinks and yellow-based shades. Test on your inside wrist before buying.

Eyes. Emphasise their beautiful almond shape by blending black or grey shadow at the outer corner of the lid. And repeat again as a socket line, blending well with a lighter lid colour (pearl shades look lovely). Kohl pencil inside the lower lid line brings out the eye shape – especially when teamed with a thin liner outside lashes and extended at the corners.

Cheeks. Blusher gives definition to cheekbones and adds shape to face. Apply with a bushy brush just below cheekbones, working out to hairline. Blusher on temples will add warmth to face. Choose a blusher with soft red tones.

Lips. Go for any shade which suits you – reds and burgundies, even a shocking pink for parties.

Fair sensitive skins

Together with red hair and freckles these sum up Celtic origins. Protection is the key word for freckly, fair skin, both from the sun and cold. Moisturisers and bases containing sunscreens are good for this skin type. If you try to tan at all, it should be gently and slowly, so go for a tinted moisturiser for colour in summer. Avoid highly perfumed products on your skin. And use a rich night cream to combat dryness.

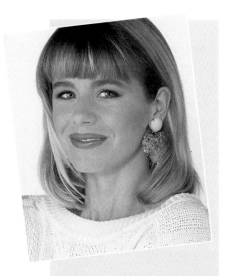

Base. Strong red and yellow tones are common to this skin type. Choose a base without pink in it because it makes any redness appear worse. Freckles form as specks of excess melanin in the skin and are charming beauty assets. But if you wish to cover them, counteract redness with a green moisturiser first and use a thick foundation with yellow or beige tones matched to your palest skin tone. An off-white powder will set the base while helping to tone down redness.

Eyebrows. Shape with a brown eyebrow pencil or powder if they're weak or fair.

Eyes. Autumnal shades, browns, golds and yellows, are lovely warm colours for redheads, but keep greens and blues to a minimum. Pinks can be worn on eyes but need to be carefully blended to avoid a harsh look. Choose brown or black mascara to define eyelashes.

Cheeks. A dusting of peachy blusher is all you'll need as your skin provides plenty of natural colour.

Lips. Deep reds and pinks look great. They'll look even better if you outline them first with a deeper shade of liner.

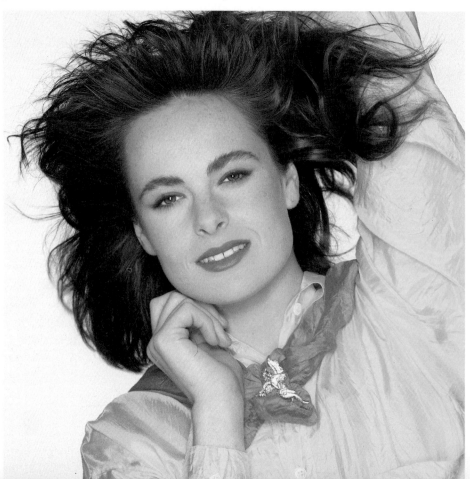

First make-ups

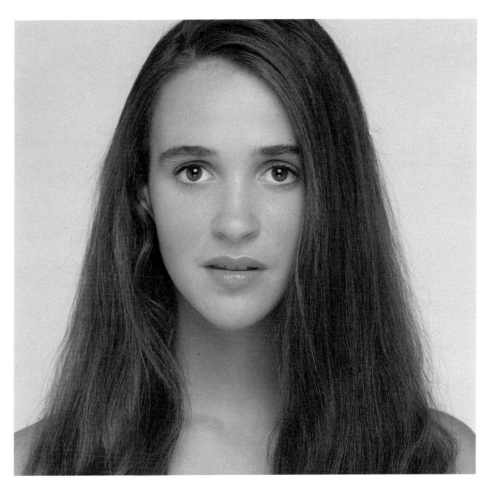

Little girls often want to experiment with make-up. By learning the basics, along with how to clean, freshen and moisturise skin, they can start to build up a good basis for later make-up looks.

Young skin, especially at puberty when it may be suffering the effects of hormonal changes, is best left alone. Apart from cleaning and moisturising, if necessary, a foundation won't add beauty. Medicated concealers can help disguise blemishes on special occasions and tinted moisturisers may bring a bloom to an extra pale young skin without giving it too much heavy cover.

The best eye basic for a first make-up is a waterproof mascara. Older teenagers may find that a hint of natural-coloured shadow (rose, beige) looks lovely for special occasions.

Avoid blushers on young faces; they'll look too heavy.

Lip colour looks much too elaborate for a first make-up. Natural tinted lipgloss helps protect lips and give a hint of shade.

There is nothing more unflattering than a young-looking face wearing too much colour. It detracts from natural freshness. Although girls of 12 onwards may wish to try out the suggestions above, save brighter, more made-up looks until late teens or twenties. When ready to take on a more made-up look, keep foundation light to allow the youthful bloom to show through or, instead, try a glowing tinted powder to shape and add colour to your face – brush over cheekbones, eyelids, tip of chin and sides of forehead. Start with subtle eye colours (browns, soft mauves, pinks, dull gold and smoky shades); heavy lines will give a painted doll effect. Young lips look best with just a hint of colour: use a soft pink, coral or a gold shade which flatters your natural lips rather than disguises them.

Older make-up looks

As you get older, your skin, like your hair, loses some of its colour (the exception being people who live in hot countries or sunbathe often when the melanin stays for longer in the skin as skin renewal slows down with age). So match your foundation accordingly, reviewing it at least every three years, and never try to compensate with a darker shade which will look false. You will also find that as fine lines and wrinkles form, your skin can't hold very heavy foundation and powder. It will gather into the smile lines and show them up more. The answer is to go for a lighter matt cover and translucent powder that stops shine but doesn't add further pigment. Remember to take foundation down past your jawline to blend in with your neck.

Eyes, too, can look ghoulish with elaborate make-up at a later age. Steer clear of shadows with too much white in them. Use a fine covering of a deeper pigmented powder which glides on well. Try using just two near-matching shades, one to cover lid and brow, the darker shade to emphasise a subtle creaseline above the existing one. Make sure eye make-up goes up towards the brow at outer corners as the brow muscle begins to sag as we get older giving a downward effect – upswept colour can counteract this. Give eyelashes one cover of a non-build-up mascara. Comb through if they look too heavy. Use a pencil to gently stroke in soft brown or grey eyebrow hairs if they are sparse.

Blusher should be confined to just around cheeks from hairline to under outer eye. Lines across the face are fine for definition on younger, line-free skins, but when you have natural lines it's best to play down the emphasis on them.

Lipstick can be tricky, as fine wrinkling around the mouth persuades it to 'bleed' into them. Stick to more subtle, softer shades which will blend with skin tone more easily and use a harder pencil (soften the lead or applicator under hot running water) to make your outline. Be sure that you lift the line a little over the natural outline at the outside corners of the top lip to counteract the unflattering down-at-mouth look.

Stick to softer, more subtle colours throughout and remember that, as your hair and skin shades change, some colours that you've always felt unflattering may now suit you, and vice versa. Try soft dusky mauve, brown, pale rose or beige eye shades, a paler baby pink blusher, lips in pale coral, strawberry or rose shades. Stick to matt colours – any shine, pearl or sparkle will highlight creases and lines.

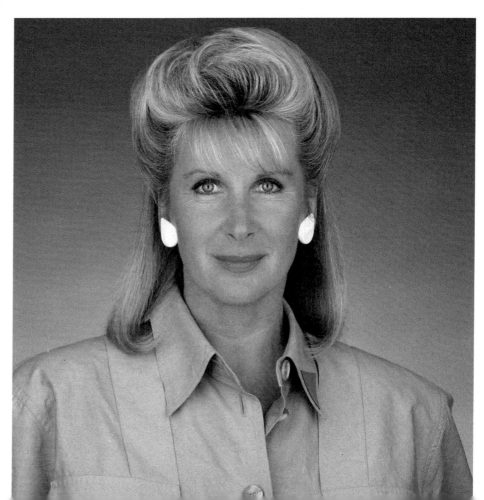

Allergy to cosmetics

This is common as they contain pigments and most have preservatives and perfume ingredients too – all high allergens for those susceptible. If you do become allergic, stop using cosmetics on that particular area immediately and if it doesn't clear up within a day or so, visit your GP. Patch test all the products used on the site of allergy on your inside arm (for eyes, for instance: cleanser, moisturiser, foundation, powders and mascara). If a reaction occurs, you will know by eliminating one at a time which particular product to avoid. However, this isn't foolproof, as skin on your eyelid, for example, is more delicate and may react to substances that will not affect other skin. It may also be that the mixture of two or more products in cleansing or blending is causing the irritating cocktail. Alternatively the allergy may be a one-off, and suddenly appear or disappear. An allergy clinic can attempt to isolate an allergen for you but it is a long process. If you suffer regularly, consider hypo-allergenic products which contain no perfume or preservatives and cut down, or out, known allergens.

Make up to the environment

IN THE SUN

No one is suggesting that sunbathers or those on holiday must wear make-up, but if you find yourself outdoors in a sunny environment and want to wear make-up, here are some tips:

Make-up can serve as a light sunscreen in sunshine. Anything with pigment in it protects your skin to some degree from the sun's rays. Of course, a sunscreen is more effective against burning (see Chapter 7, Sunbathing) but as a base it will make your skin greasier and make-up on top more likely to melt. Your skin provides its own greasy layer of sweat – an oil and water mixture – when it's hot, and although this isn't a sunscreen sweat is protective and antibacterial. But it is disastrous for oil-based cosmetics. You should stick, instead, to powders that absorb it or gel- or water-based cosmetics that sink into your skin.

Foundations tend to run and crease with heat and sweat. Instead, use a tinted moisturiser which gives skin a good protective seal to stop it dehydrating while allowing perspiration to escape. The pigment sinks into the skin to give an even skintone. Alternatively a fake tan product will tint skin for a week or so (see Fake Tan section, Chapter 7) so you don't need any other skin colour. If your face is inclined to flush in the heat, use a green or mauve base under your foundation.

Blushers should look cool rather than rosy in the heat and cream ones can melt, so stay with natural or soft powder shades. Some emollient powder formulas are waterproof and smudgeproof.

Eyes. An eye-fix primer will give double staying power if it's used under a powder shadow. Some shadows claim that they're creaseproof and contain a binder to seal in colour and help prevent creasing. Waterproof mascaras are usually heatproof, too.

Lips. Any glossy lipstick will smudge over your lipline in hot weather. Longer lasting formulas usually leave colour when the gloss goes; the darker the shade, the stronger the stain. Prepare lips first with a primer. Line lips with a strong, non-smudgy pencil in a shade similar to the lipstick, then blot with a tissue, dust with powder and fill in with long-lasting lipstick.

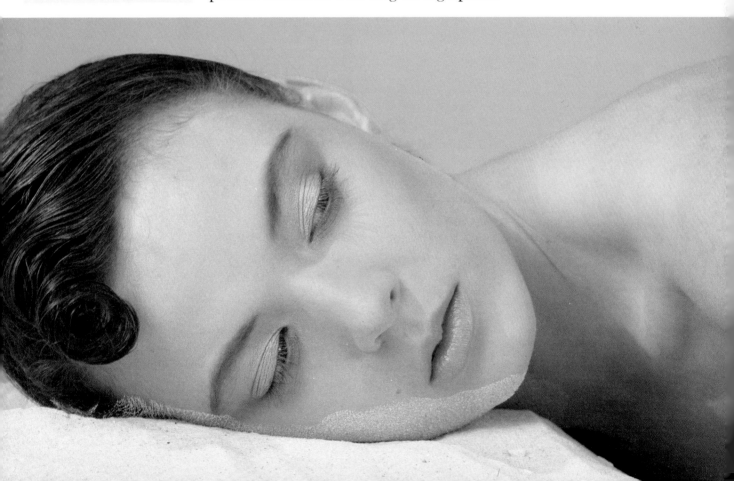

IN THE WATER

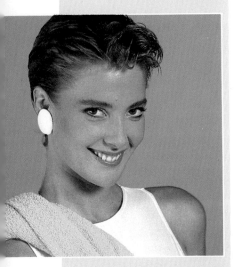

And this means from a downpour to a swimming pool! If you feel you need some colour, here's how to choose non-dissoluble ones. Waterproof make-up needs oil to deflect the water and allow the tint to stay on your skin. 'Long-lasting' does not mean 'waterproof', though sometimes products are both. To be 'waterproof' a product must stay on the skin after a dip – though that doesn't allow for rubbing eyes, heat or creasing.

Foundation. A water-based one will streak; so choose a water-in-oil-emulsion (a thicker emulsion) to stay on in most wet conditions. A waterproof tinted sunscreen will even up skintone and give a hint of colour while swimming in the sun.

Blushers. Stick or cream blushers will stay on in water though they melt in heat. There are waterproof powder blushers with an emollient formula which have staying power, too.

Eyes. Pencils are oil based, and fine for water. Choose a colour to match your costume. There are many waterproof mascaras, mainly because eyes water! To be non-flaky they also need emollient properties. Apply mascara to well blotted, non-moisturised lashes.

Lips. A fine lipgloss in a natural shade or long-lasting lipstick will also stay on in water.

FOR STAYING POWER

When time is short and you need looks to last, try these:

Moisturise at least an hour before applying long-lasting make-up so moisturiser is absorbed into the skin.

Keep cool when you put on make-up. Apply it in a cool, dry atmosphere to dry skin for maximum staying power.

Look out for long-lasting cosmetic ranges or products in brands which say they give extra staying power. An oil-based product tends to run after a few hours whereas powders fade and don't show up so badly if they smudge. Use paler more natural shades so that the fading away will be less noticeable. Eye and lip primers and fixers are made especially for giving lasting power to make-up. Put them under or over your make-up (whichever applies to the product), and allow to sink in (test with fingertip) before applying more make-up.

Set make-up with water spray. For evenings, brush on a final dusting of loose or translucent powder.

Forget about mascara by dyeing your lashes. Go to a qualified beautician or do it at home with an eyelash dye kit from a chemist.

Rinse-off cleansers aren't going to work well on waterproof make-up which shouldn't wash off with water! You'll need a greasy cleanser. Remove waterproof mascara with products made especially for it.

If you have a few minutes to spare throughout the day why not build up a basic morning face? Start with a tinted moisturiser or light foundation, pale powder eyeshadow, a soft smudge of pencil liner, minimum blusher and lipstick. For a smarter look, pat over face (especially eyes) with tissue after smudging away creases of colour on eyelids. Then add a foundation and translucent powder, blotting it into the face. Add two powder shades to eyes and strengthen the liner and then mascara. Draw a lip line and paint in lipstick, blot, powder and re-apply. For a more glittery evening look, simply add another lipstick in a stronger colour. Dust temples with a coppery or pearly shade after reinforcing blusher. And emphasise eyes more by adding extra liner and a highlighter on centre lid and browbone.

LIGHTING EFFECTS

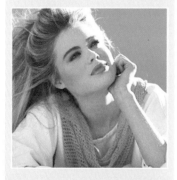

Which light you're making up for – be it day, fluorescent or spotlight – should influence the type of cosmetics you use. Follow this guide:

Daylight

This shows up everything, and that includes all skin or make-up faults. So make-up must be precise and perfect. The colours should be subtle, well blended and complement each other. Stand in front of a window and use a magnifying mirror when making up for day, to be sure you don't overdo it.

Base. Look at your skin tones in daylight for shades of pink or yellow and choose a base to match. Test foundation on your face rather than your neck which is often a different colour. Set it to last with a fine translucent powder brushed over foundation to stop it melting into your skin.

Cheeks. Just a little blusher will be enough to give you a healthy glow in daylight. Blend your blusher in with a bushy brush, avoiding harsh slabs and wedge shapes which can look artificial in clear light.

Eyes should not be weighed down with dark, heavy colours or hardened by harsh lines. Soften by using paler shades and blending

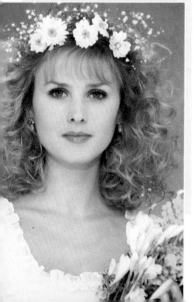

eye make-up well. Layer your shadow, blending it with cotton wool buds to keep it in place longer. Curl your lashes with an eyelash curler and use minimum mascara to stop lashes looking too spiky.

Lips. Cover lips with foundation before applying lipstick to make it longer lasting. Prevent lipstick bleeding by outlining lips with a lip pencil in the same shade as your lipstick. Or use a pale lipstick which gradually wears off without showing smudges.

Fluorescent light

Basically a cold white light with a greenish tinge to it, and this makes it harsh on make-up. The same UV light is used in discos, where it picks up glowing, white clothes, teeth and even dandruff! Steer clear of make-up that's too sparkly and stick to strong pigments with less white in them to bring life to your face.

Base. Choose a shade darker than that of your normal base. It will help you lose that washed-out look, which this light tends to create. And don't forget to put it all over your face and neck. A dusting of matt powder (not translucent, it will glow!) will set your base and give a velvety finish to your skin.

Cheeks. Try a cream blusher, over base and under powder, dotted along top of cheekbones then gently blended in with fingertips.

Eyes. Blend matt shadow into your outer lid towards the temple. Sparkly or pearl shadows all over lids will stand out too much but a dot in the centre of the top lid, applied over make-up, will open eyes up.

Lips. Rich deep dark shades will bring warmth to your face under fluorescent light. Steer clear of blue-pinks which tend to look cold.

Spotlight

In the right place spotlight can be flattering but it has to be very carefully positioned to give the desired look. When wrong, spotlights can give you deep dark sockets for eyes. Put your face in front of a table lamp with the shade removed when making up for spotlight.

Base. First apply a light concealer on under-eye shadows. Then even out skin tone with smooth flawless base. Go for matt, natural looking foundation and finish off with a translucent powder. Make sure you don't miss any areas with your foundation – it will show immediately.

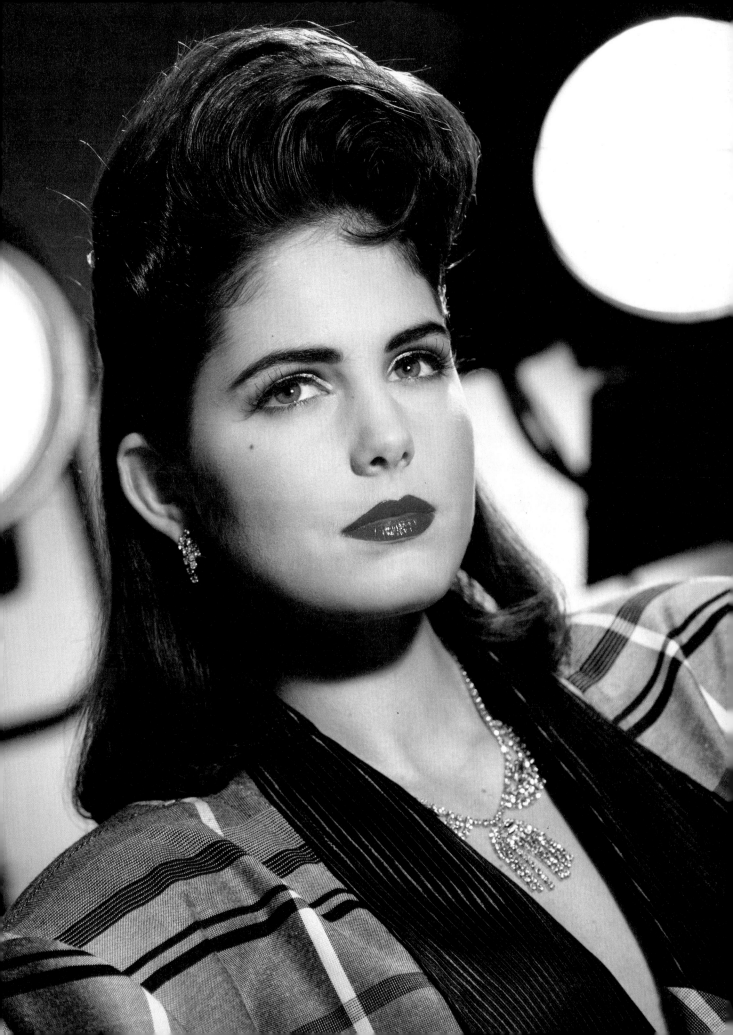

Cheeks. Blusher brings warmth to the face and is important to your appearance under a spotlight. So choose a colour from looking at your skin tones and then shade cheekbones and temples well.

Eyes. Shimmery shades show up well in spotlight – soft bright colours flatter pale eyes, stronger colours are good for dark ones. Define with eyeliner, across top lids with an upward movement at outer corners to make eyes appear wider. An eyelash comb will separate lashes after you've applied mascara.

Lips. Make the most of your mouth with a deep or bright lipstick. Add a pale highlighter on the centre of the lower lip to catch the light and make it look fuller.

Special party effects

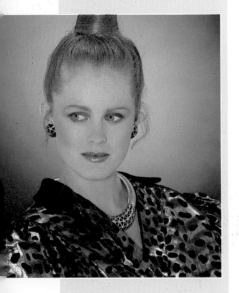

Here are some tricks and tips for taking a basic make-up look that bit further for parties:

- Try white eye pencil inside bottom lashes as kohl – it makes the eyes look wider. Alternatively, a pale pearly shade gives extra eye appeal.

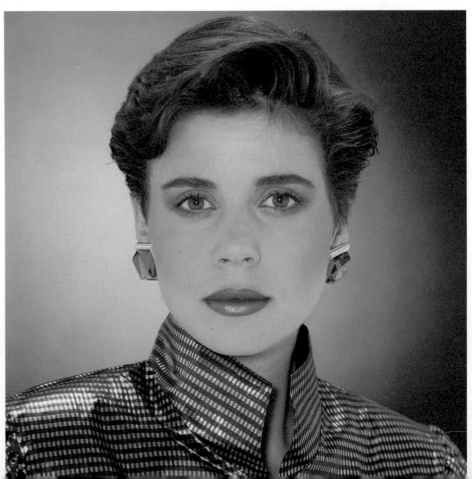

Match make-up to jewellery – be it gold, copper or silver.

Add a sprinkle of fine gold dust to cheekbones, chin, centre lids, forehead and hair so you glimmer in the light – carry on down to your shoulders, top arms, cleavage and shins for an all-over effect.

Paint your mascara through your eyebrows – even if it's coloured.

Put a touch of gold or silver shadow on the tips of blacked eyelashes.

Get glossy with a lipgloss to make lips look extra pouty.

Mix shadows to get the colours you'd like: pink and blue make mauve – you'll get the right shade by experimenting and it's easier than searching for one in the shops.

Paint eyeliner in dots for extra wide eye definition, then fill in the spaces with a bright pink or mauve.

Budget beauty

You can cut the cost of cosmetics with a little forethought. Here's how to economise on your beauty buys:

Don't throw away last year's shades. They often come back into fashion a year or so later – sometimes for different areas. There's no reason why last year's pale pink eye highlight shouldn't be next year's over or under eye colour.

Blend pearly colours – they can lighten a matt eye or lip shade – or try petroleum jelly to make lipsticks more glossy and lighter. Mix shades together with a brush or on your face to make a brand new colour.

Double or triple up. Just because a pencil is sold as an eyeliner, there's no reason why it can't become a lip liner, eyebrow pencil or kohl. A mid-brown pencil will do all these. Pinks, reds, rusts, creams and golds can be used as lipstick, blusher or eye shades. Concealer used to lighten under-eye shadows or hide blemishes makes a good highlighter along the top of cheeks or browbones; or, dotted on eyelid or lip, concealers can be used for shaping and highlighting.

Use the last bit of your lipstick or stick eyeshade by investing in a fine-tipped brush to reach the stub below the container line. A fine brush will also reach the edges of hardened powder in a palette; you can dampen the brush with water to paint it on or use it as a liner. Keep old mascara brushes and use a longer one to reach the last bit of mascara at the bottom of the tube.

Hold skincare jars and bottles under hot water to soften and bring away the last dab.

Tacky remains of nail polishes will become fluid again when you add a few drops of remover and shake.

CHAPTER 5
_____

Setting Style

However clever you are with make-up it won't look good if it's inappropriate to your individual style and the surroundings you're wearing it in. That goes for clothes and accessories, too. What may look great on someone else can look unflattering on you or, equally, a stunning get-up for a club or party is often totally wrong for a wedding or at work. So, as important as learning the ground rules for general good looks is assessing and putting into practice what suits you and your environment. The careful marriage of all these ingredients goes towards making you look and feel comfortable, self-confident and attractive.

Your own style

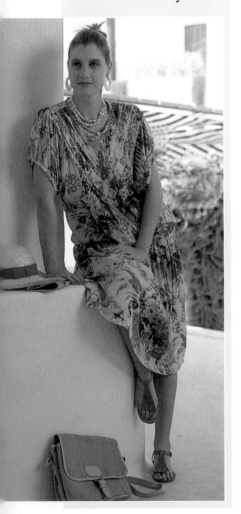

Switching your style to your mood is fun – become a country girl with minimum or no make-up and jewellery in a casual tracksuit, or a sexy siren with a dressed-up look, dark eyes and close-fitting clothes. Knowing what you *don't* look good in is just as important. Some people, for instance, just aren't glitter types: they won't look or feel good with sparkle on their faces or bodies. Others don't suit deep lipstick shades, elaborate eye make-up, earrings, high heels or trousers. Finding out what does and doesn't suit you is the trickiest but most enjoyable part of good looks. One of your best beauty bonuses is an honest and critical good friend. Better than mothers, who usually see their daughters as little girls in pigtails with scrubbed faces, or partners who will sometimes decide a 'natural'-looking wife is preferable to someone who might catch another man's eye, a friend whose taste you admire and who isn't inclined to jealousy can give you honest comment on new clothes, make-up and hairstyles.

Otherwise learn from visual aids: copy looks that you admire in magazines, but first be sure that the model is similar to you: check her colouring, age, face shape, figure or whatever is relevant. Keep up to date with beauty and fashion features in magazines: new looks need not be expensive, more a matter of noticing what is fashionable. Bring yourself up to date by matching different separates and colours together, changing your heel height or belt width or tucking a sweater in or pulling it out. Borrow jewellery and accessories from friends to see if they suit you – and if you're not sure, try out new looks gradually to see if you feel comfortable and to gauge the reaction of others.

Suit your surroundings

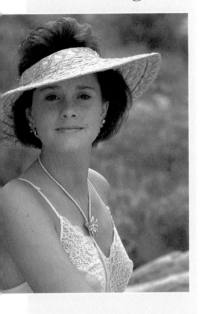

Now you've found your individual style, learn to apply it. First be practical. Will it be cold? Will you be walking far? Will you get windswept? Do you need to wear something that doesn't crease from sitting? Be appropriate too – a plunge neckline might be fine for friends but not in an office or when seeing elderly relatives; dramatic make-up is great for a night out but not for a country weekend, and it can look odd when you're going to the local shops. If you're not one who likes to stand out in a crowd, find out what kind of look others will be wearing; and then ask for details. Does casual mean your oldest jeans, a tracksuit or just not dressed up? Does an evening dress mean that it has to be long? Some old-fashioned restaurants still won't allow in women wearing trousers – even if they're made of silk and part of a stunning outfit. On the other hand you may feel totally overdressed in the same outfit at a local bistro. With a bit of research and some sensible forethought, you can always feel comfortable and look your best.

Suit all the senses

The hidden ingredient to beauty is the way you smell. Perfume is one of the most alluring and mysterious beauty assets – so long as you choose one that suits your character and chemistry. The perfume world is shrouded in intrigue, its manufacturers using aspirational words that hint at luxury. The word perfume comes from the Latin *par fumum* which means 'through the smoke'. This is because originally resins and balms were burnt as incense to release their fragrance.

A master perfumer creates new fragrances for perfume houses and is called a 'nose'. Great noses are born with the talent of being able to finely differentiate between smells. Their odour memories, developed through experience, allow them to judge how different essences will react together and create an attractive blend of smells for popular use. This traditional art is still very much alive and even in this technological age is almost ritualistic. The perfumer's workplace is known as the fragrance organ, the materials being arranged around him or her in tiers like organ pipes ready to hand for the nose to start smelling and mixing.

Any one fragrance can contain between 20 and 300 raw materials – some synthetic, some extracts from fruits, flowers, herbs, animal secretions and so on. That said, most perfumes in the shops today will fit into one of seven perfume families:

Florals are the most popular and largest group. The fragrance may conjure up the essence of one flower or a general floral bouquet.

Aldehydes are synthetic materials which aim to give a smoky type of aroma. These are considered ultra feminine!

Chypre combine mossy smelling essences with fresh citrus. So they're soft with a surprising tang.

Greens are the fresh country air fragrances reminiscent of grass, leaves, stems and meadows.

Orientals tend to be sweet and heavy, like exotic Eastern blossoms.

Tobacco, leather are synthetic and masculine, with aromas suggestive of their names.

Fougère are also masculine and combine the herbal scent of lavender with a mossy foundation.

Various families may be combined into a single 'note'. Notes are the impressions of each aroma which make up a whole perfume. The life of a perfume is usually divided into three notes:

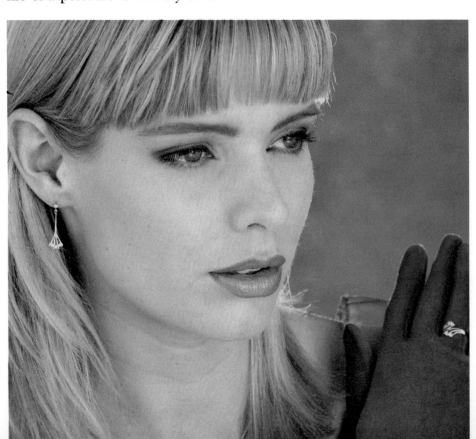

The top note is the first impression you get from a perfume and the first to fade after application.

The middle note is the core of the perfume which gains definition from the warmth and chemistry of the wearer's skin.

The base note is the longest lasting part of the perfume and the one which gradually fades after a few hours.

Manufacturers 'fix' their perfumes with materials which help to slow down evaporation and make the scent last longer. But the life of a perfume on your skin also depends on the strength you buy. These vary in different perfume houses but as a broad guide:

Perfume or Extrait is the strongest, containing 15–30 per cent perfume oils and 70 per cent alcohol.

Parfum de toilette, Eau de parfum or Esprit de parfum contain 8–15 per cent perfume oil to around 85 per cent alcohol.

Eau de toilette is made with around 6 per cent perfume oil to 80 per cent alcohol and water to lighten the fragrance.

Eau de cologne is a solution of around 3–5 per cent perfume oil in an alcohol and water mix. It contains only a few fixing ingredients so is refreshing rather than long-lasting.

When buying a perfume always wait at least four to six hours after trying and before buying to find out if you like the three notes and how long it takes to fade. Make sure you are warm when testing; perfume doesn't develop fully on cold skin. You may find the more expensive perfume more economical in the long run than a cheaper Eau de toilette, as you use less and it lasts for longer on the skin. But remember that the greasier your skin the more diluted the perfume will be and the more quickly it will wear away. Dry skins tend to hold scent on them for longer, and perfume smells different on different skins and at different times. For instance, if you've been drinking alcohol or eating spicy foods, in hot weather or during times of hormonal activity, perfume will mingle with perspiration and create a different scent. Apply perfume to warm pulse spots for maximum effect: behind ears, at base of neck, between breasts, on wrists. And make sure it's not fighting for attention with your deodorant or hairspray.

Aftershaves and men's colognes are perfumes for men. More men are now making themselves smell nice with added scent, and manufacturers are reflecting this by introducing many new lines of toiletries and colognes, including scented lotions for soothing skin and bodycare products.

CHAPTER 6

Shape Up

So you want a different shape?

The bad news first: you can't change your proportions drastically except by radical cosmetic surgery (and sometimes not even then – see Chapter 9). If you've got a big bust, hips or thighs compared to the rest of you, it'll always be that way. Weight loss may appear to go from one area (especially the skinnier parts of you – perhaps your face or breasts) but dieting causes an overall loss, rather than in just one spot. And there's not much point in losing inches when it leaves you with flabby, wobbly flesh. The answer is to exercise. Along with good posture, it's wise to think about the benefits of exercise whether or not you're slimming but it's especially important when you're losing weight and need to firm up.

Posture

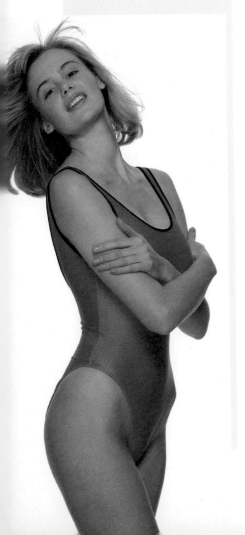

The first step to a good shape and the basis to all exercise is good posture. Finding out how to balance and hold your body frame helps even out pressure on bones and organs as well as on the digestive track and prevents problems that extra weight on those areas could cause. Problems such as arthritis, headaches and backache can be considerably eased by finding a good way of evenly distributing your weight. Good posture also makes you look slimmer and a better, neater shape while showing a sense of confidence and ease with your body.

Taller people are more prone to sloping their shoulders and craning their necks in an effort to become less conspicuous and nearer the average height. Shorter people usually have good posture as they often stretch their spines in an effort to add some inches to their height. Check which you do by trying to catch sight of yourself 'unposed' in a mirror when you're standing normally. Better still, use a double mirror so that you can see your back and side views, too – for instance, in a department store's changing room.

The best standing position. Place feet pointing forwards, about a foot apart, with weight balanced equally on each foot and knees relaxed but not bent. Leave hands and arms hanging loosely at your sides. Now imagine a string pulling you up from the top of your head, making your spine stretch. At the same time relax shoulders down and back, and pull your stomach and bottom up and in (towards each other). Now you have found the correct way to stand

– try to slip into this position each time you are standing still.

The worst standing position is with one knee bent and all your weight on the other leg, your shoulders tilted and hand on hip.

The best walking posture. Using the standing posture, try to move smoothly from the thigh/hip joint, putting your heel down first and breathing deeply and regularly. If you often carry heavy shopping or a briefcase, try to disperse the weight into two bags or alternate carrying hands and wear lower heels for longer walks. Remember to keep your head up when you walk.

The worst walking posture is head down, with shuffling steps putting toes down first so you kick up dirt.

The best sitting position is with hips in the direction that you're looking and thighs pointed forwards, pulling your stomach in, stretching spine and, if possible, supported upright by the back of the chair. Relax shoulders and put feet flat on the floor. Bend forwards from the hips rather than rounding your spine to reach out.

The worst sitting position is leaning heavily on one arm of the chair with your arm supporting your weight and legs crossed or your feet under you on the seat. Slumped backwards with the weight supported on the area of your spine between your shoulder blades on the back of your chair is also bad posture.

Driving. Try a sitting position with arms out as far as possible to reach the steering wheel (while comfortably able to reach the pedals with your feet).

Bending. Always bend at the knees, keeping back straight.

Lying. Try to keep your spine straight and legs as straight as possible. Too high pillows in bed can curve the spine and hinder easy breathing.

Exercise

Now that your resting and everyday movements are aligned, think about firming up your silhouette. Exercise strengthens the muscles and ligaments that hold flesh to your bones and so makes them tauter to your skeletal frame. It builds up those muscles that define your overall shape (but doesn't necessarily make your shape more muscly if you control exercise carefully). The good news is that you can work on specific areas with exercise, to tone and firm them and make these parts a better shape. But you will always have to work hard on these areas to keep them like this. However, the areas of fatty nodules called cellulite are a different type of problem; gentle exercise may help, but not solve, the dimpled skin here (see cellulite section later in this chapter).

If you're happy with your weight but feel that exercise will help you shape up – you may find that after a while although you still look as slim, the scales register a heavier weight. This is because you are turning fat to muscle and muscle weighs more. Many athletes have less body fat but weigh more than most of us.

Exercise has the added advantage of taking blood away from the digestive track and into the muscles doing the work. For this reason, it can lessen appetite. It also means you should not exercise directly after a meal when your system should be concentrating on digesting food; instead, plan exercise or sport sessions for at least an hour after eating or better still just before the next meal. Being active gets the metabolism going, pushing oxygen around the body faster to feed new cells and get rid of used waste matter. With the right planning, it'll help your eyes shine, your skin glow, make you feel fitter and supply you with more energy.

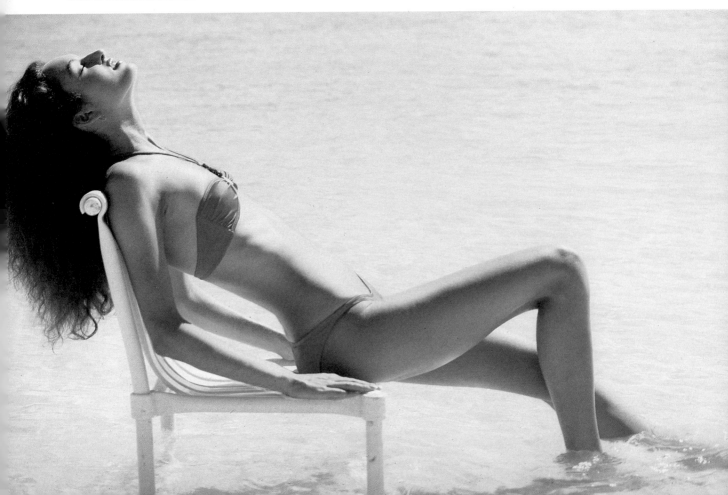

Much worse than not taking enough exercise, is doing it too rigorously. There are hospitals full of people with sporting injuries – ranging from slipped discs and sprained joints to deep bruising and fractures. You should never shoot out of bed into a hectic exercise session. Muscles need to be eased and warmed up properly. And if you've recently been ill or had a baby, are pregnant or have heart problems, consult your doctor before doing *any* type of exercise.

WARM-UP

If you watch a dog or cat rousing from sleep for a spot of activity, they nearly always get up slowly and stretch. Humans can benefit from watching our clever furry friends. The best way to start a warm-up is lying on your back on a firm but soft covering or mat, but anywhere that you can relax will do. Start at the tips of your toes and, moving up to your ankles and calves, stretch each part of your body in turn until you reach the top of your head. Then jog gently on the spot or go for a walk for ten minutes. Now you're ready to exercise.

SPOT EXERCISE
Breasts and upper arms
Stand up straight, with arms bent and fingertips just touching under your chin. Keep forearms at shoulder level and pull elbows back as far as you can, breathing out each time you pull. Do 10, relax arms, then 10 more.

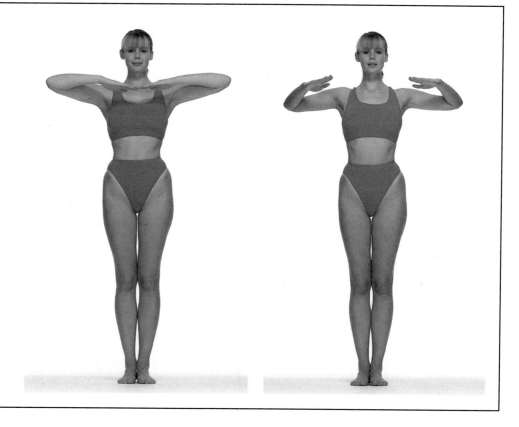

Waist

Stand with feet about a foot apart. Put your arms up straight and, bending wrists, clasp fingers over your head. Keeping back straight, bend to the side as far as you can go, as you breathe out. Return upright as you breathe in and do the same bend to the other side as you breathe out again. Do 10 bends on each side.

Now place feet further apart and put arms straight out from shoulders. Keeping arms and legs straight, bend and twist from the waist to touch left foot with your right hand as you breathe out. Breathe in as you return to starting position and repeat on the other side. Do 10 on each side.

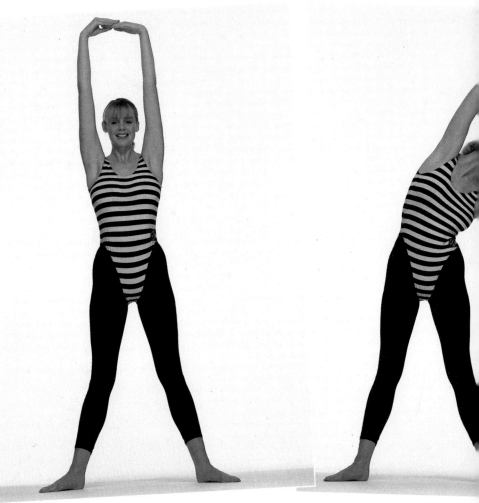

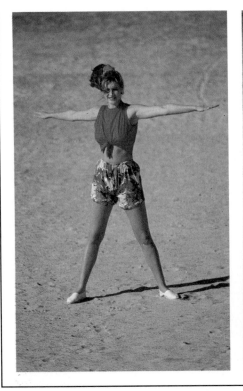

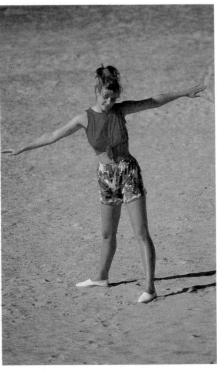

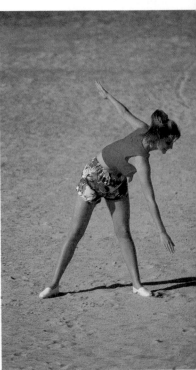

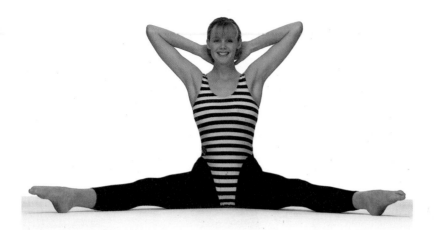

Now sit on the floor with your legs straight out and apart. Clasp hands behind your head and twist to try to touch right knee with left elbow as you breathe out. Breathe in as you return to sitting position and repeat on the other side. Repeat 10 times.

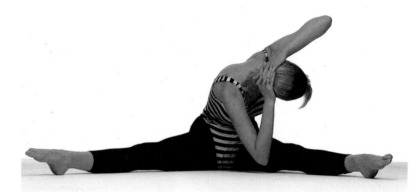

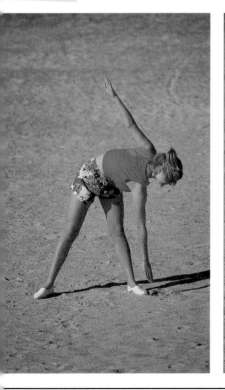
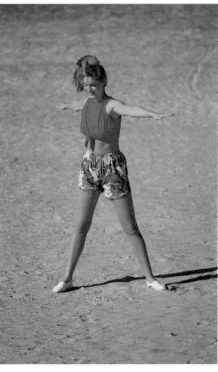
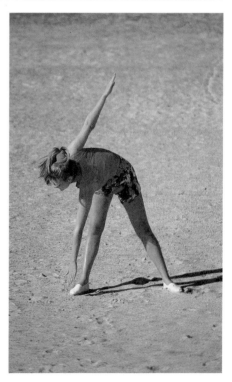

Stomach

Lie on your back with legs straight out and together, toes pointed. As you breathe out, lift one leg about a foot from the floor and circle five times with your toes in the air. Breathe in as you circle five times in the other direction, then lower leg. Repeat with the other leg.

Bottom and thighs

Stand up straight with feet together, sideways to a wall and supporting yourself against it with your hand. Keeping leg straight, point the toe furthest away from the wall and swing your leg up as far in front of you as it will go as you breathe out; then breathe in as you swing it back behind you. Swing 20 times and repeat with other leg (facing the other way).

Legs

Stand up straight with feet together and put arms straight out in front of you (as though sleepwalking). Rise up on tiptoes as you breathe in, then slowly breathe out as you bend at the knees, gradually going down as far as you can, remembering to keep back straight. Breathe in as you slowly raise yourself again. Try doing this 10 times.

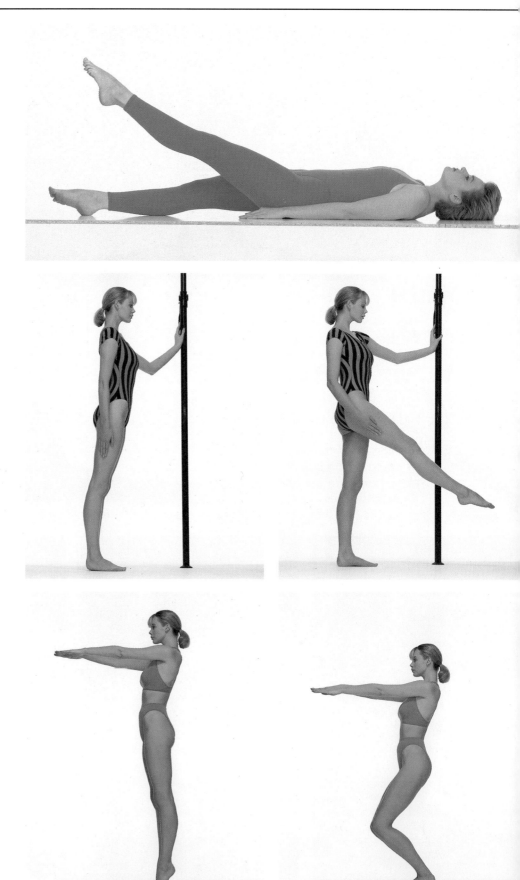

NB. You can build up
these exercises and do
more as you get fitter
and more supple.

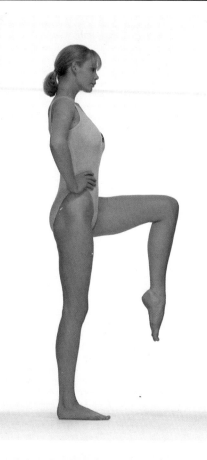

Calves

Stand up straight with
feet together and hands
on hips. Lift right knee
until thigh is at
right-angles to your body
(lower leg and toe
pointing down) as you
breathe in. Now breathe
out as you rotate lower
leg, drawing circles in
the air with your toes.
Change direction after
five circles as you
breathe in and do five
more. Now lower leg
slowly as you breathe out
and repeat with the other
leg.

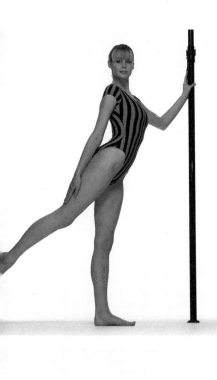

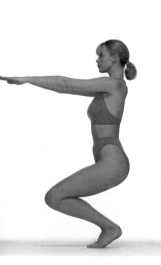

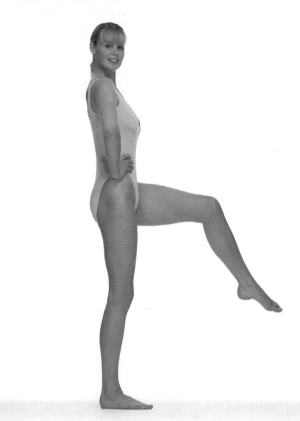

WATER EXERCISES

Apart from swimming, which is one of the best exercises (see next section), water is an excellent medium in which to do specific exercises. Callisthenics, as they are known, are ideal for those who swim regularly or enjoy poolside or beach holidays. The buoyancy helps relieve some of those muscles we use every day on dry land (in feet and legs) while movement and water pressure can be used to exercise other less active muscles.

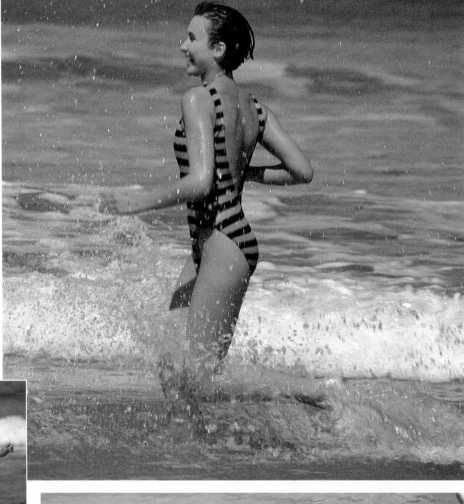

Running through the waves
Puts pressure on the thighs as lower legs are pushed against the water.

Jumping the waves
Good for hip joint, thighs and bottom.

Kicks
Hold on to the bar or edge of the pool lying on your stomach and, keeping legs as straight as possible, kick out of the water – good for stomach, legs and bottom.

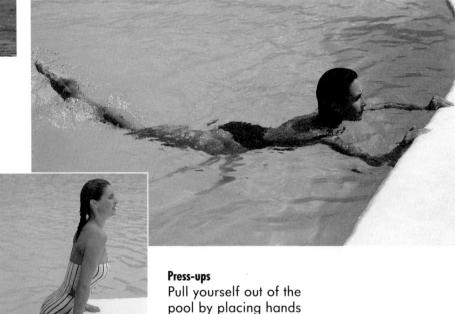

Press-ups
Pull yourself out of the pool by placing hands flat on the side and lifting your body. Firms shoulders and arms.

SPORT

Sports provide excellent exercise and have the added advantage of being fun. The activity often becomes a social occasion, and sometimes takes place outside in oxygen-giving, healthy fresh air. Some sports tone up certain parts of the body particularly while others give all-over benefits and can be a good way of firming up generally before you embark on something more strenuous. So choose a sport to suit you. Here is a guide to gentle sports and exercise, medium ones for the fit and strenuous sports for the extra fit and flexible.

GENTLY DOES IT

The following sports or exercises will give you all-over body toning and can be taken slowly to begin with then built up as you feel more fit.

Walking. 3 to 5 calories used per minute. Is now considered, along with swimming, one of the best exercises you can do. Try to walk instead of getting the bus or going up or down in a lift, and aim to take half an hour to an hour's walking exercise each day, outside in a relaxed atmosphere, while breathing deeply and evenly. If you haven't got a dog borrow one and do it a favour, too!

Swimming. 5–15 calories used per minute. The gravity free properties of water give muscles that don't usually work a chance to exercise while relaxing those that you use a lot (especially feet and legs). For maximum benefit aim to swim at least three times a week for half an hour. And if you don't know how, learn at your local pool – it'll be just as good for you.

Tennis. 6–8 calories used per minute. A good all round sport if you play someone of the same ability.

Exercises particularly the arms, shoulders, waist and legs.

Bowling. 3–5 calories used per minute. Exercises waist and arms.

Horseriding. 3–10 calories used per minute. Exercises legs, thighs, bottom, arms and shoulders.

Table Tennis. 2–8 calories used per minute. Exercises arms, shoulders, waist – and legs.

Cycling. 4–15 calories used per minute. Good for toning legs and bottom.

Golf. 4–7 calories used per minute. Same as walking, with better exercise for waist and shoulders while driving a shot.

Roller/Ice Skating. 5–18 calories used per minute. Good exercise for the legs and arms.

Judo/Martial Arts. 2–8 calories used per minute. Although you'll need some tuition and have to be prepared to join a club, all the martial arts provide good all-over exercise.

MEDIUM EXERTION

With these sports and exercises, it's important to warm up first and start slowly, then build up to longer sessions.

Running. 10–12 calories used per minute. Good all-over exercise. First, make sure you have good fitting running shoes. Start by running for a few minutes, then walking for a few minutes. Increase time of running

and length of run by a few minutes each day until you reach your ideal. Running every other day can be just as beneficial as running every day if you go for a walk on the days in between.

Dancing. 6–10 calories used per minute. Lively dancing (especially disco) exercises all of the body. Make the most of parties.

Skiing. 5–18 calories used per minute. It's wise to take a few lessons and exercise those muscles you'll be using before going on a skiing holiday. Good for legs, bottom and arms.

Weight Training. Tones up muscles by making them work harder. You can choose which parts of the body you tone up but it's wise to go to a qualified trainer who will advise you on which weights are right for your level of fitness.

Badminton. 6–10 calories used per minute. Good all-over exercise and available to anyone with enough room to put up a net – home kits are available in sports shops.

Basket/Netball. 7–9 calories used per minute. Good all-over exercise. Warm up and practise well before attempting a strenuous match.

Waterskiing. 3–5 calories used per minute. Exercises arms and shoulders along with thighs.

Windsurfing. 3–5 calories used per minute. Good for arms and waist. (See Swimming section if you're not very good!)

FOR THE EXTRA FIT

You should only attempt these if you're already fit and flexible. Alternatively, try to do these sports gently with breaks every few minutes, slowly building up to a long session. Never push yourself further than feels good.

Skipping. 5–7 calories used per minute. Currently the most fashionable exercise – you need to be fit to skip for any length of time. It's aerobic and similar in action to jogging.

Gymnastics. 5–12 calories used per minute. These can be started slowly but you'll need to be quite fit to do some of the exercises. Find a good trainer to advise you.

Squash. 10–18 calories used per minute. All-over exercise. Protective eye goggles are now advised.

Jogging. 10–12 calories used per minute. Good aerobic exercise. Tones up legs. Women should wear a good supportive sports bra to prevent sore nipples and correct jogging shoes are advised.

WHAT'S WHAT IN EXERCISE

Aerobic means 'with oxygen' and covers repetitive exercises such as running, swimming, cycling, skipping and so on, where you're encouraged to breathe regularly as you move. The aim is to increase circulation and lung capacity and speed up heartbeat so oxygen is delivered around the body faster. The cardiovascular system will become more effective as a result.

Isometric exercises are the opposite of aerobics and, with little movement of the rest of the body, aim to make just certain muscles work harder to tone them without moving the joints. Clenching your buttocks to tone up your bottom, pushing palms together in front of you to firm breasts are isometric exercises.

Cramp. These contracted muscles are usually caused by muscle fatigue, bad circulation or when muscles are out of condition or cold. Try stretching against the position that they have contracted into or massaging the offending area.

Sprains and strains. A sprain is a series of minute tears on an overstretched ligament (tissue that attaches one bone to another). A strain is the equivalent on a muscle tendon (which attaches muscles to bone). If you're susceptible to these, a support wrap or brace can help protect you from further damage. Experts believe that cold packs applied immediately after the injury reduce pain, swelling and haemorrhaging (use a cold sponge or ice wrapped in a towel).

CELLULITE

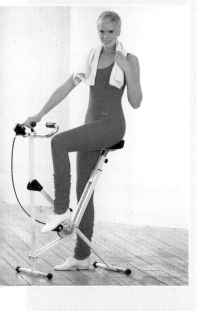

Some British doctors don't believe it exists – anyone who's got it or has even seen it is sure that it does! Cellulite is the dimpled, orange-peel-like skin that forms anywhere from the breast to the region of the knee but usually around hips, bottoms and thighs. Men don't have it – they may have pot bellies and flabby figures but only women are unlucky enough to suffer from the dimpled effect. This is why these clumps of fat with added water are thought to be hormonally induced and related to fluid retention. Cellulite often appears at times of hormonal activity. Gentle exercise to improve circulation and avoiding water retention can help reduce cellulite. Regular massage of the offending area may help clear it a little, as will not wearing too tight clothes or becoming too overweight (though it strikes the thin as much as the more rounded, and fat can cover and disguise cellulite). But all the creams and massage treatments available won't cure it. Nor can liposuction remove it (unlike other fat cells; see Cosmetic Surgery section, Chapter 9).

EXERCISE EQUIPMENT

Bicycle and rowing machines, which ape the action of the real thing, aim to tone you up in the same way. Basically an exercise bicycle firms up legs and bottom, a rowing machine firms up waist, arms, shoulders and breasts. Weights and dumbells give isotonic exercise – with muscles and joints being exercised together. Before embarking on these, it's wise to find out how fit you are. A professional trainer at a health club or gym will be able to assess this.

What you wear is important exercise equipment. Go to a reputable sports shop for the correct fitting of a shoe especially made for the sport you're going to enjoy. For instance, joggers need soft, thick-soled training shoes to absorb some of the shock when pounding on hard surfaces. Make sure the clothes you wear aren't too tight (a leotard, for example, should allow you to feel comfortable in any position) and women, even with the smallest breasts, should wear a good supportive bra for rigorous activity.

HOW TO FIND OUT MORE ABOUT A SPORT

The Sports Council, 16 Upper Woburn Place, London WC1H 0QP, will give you a list of specific organisations if you send them a stamped, self-addressed envelope. Or your local library or town hall may have information on facilities, clubs and professional trainers in the area.

Find out how fit you are by taking your pulse then comparing it to your exercising pulse rate. Take the first rate (on your wrist at the base of your thumb) first thing in the morning before any exercise, eating or drinking. The average for men is between 70 and 85 a minute, for women between 75 and 90 a minute (the rate declines as you get older). If you are fit and fall into this category, take your pulse again after some exercise. Maximum rate is around 200 a minute for younger people, down to 175 for older people, and the exercising rate for a fit person should not be more than three-quarters of this rate. Don't worry if you don't fall within these guidelines – but do go for a check-up with your doctor.

A slimmer shape

Back in the sixties, we aspired to an anorexic Twiggy-type figure – underweight by any standards. Looking further back to the fifties, forties and thirties, most glamorous women such as Marilyn Monroe were often overweight by today's fashionable standards – but were considered ideal then and were certainly not overweight according to any weight chart guidelines. Today we're seeing something of a gradual weight revolution, and it's a healthy one. While fashionable models are still thinner than necessary, the emphasis is on finding a good shape and healthy diet rather than being too concerned about what the scales say.

Having said that, it still seems to be a big business preoccupation to 'lose a few pounds'. Fashionable clothes, slimming foods and articles on slimming all give the impression that 'slimmer is better'.

Why? Well, there is a theory that, like all beauty treatments, we do it to look better for others but it's also something we enjoy doing for ourselves. We see our 'ideal' weight as an achievement and we enjoy feeling guilty and in need of help if we cheat, or proud of our success and fashionable figure if we succeed. Like climbing mountains, some do it for the struggles and traumas of getting there! But slimming is not as dangerous as mountain climbing unless, of course, you fall into the terrible traps of bulimia nervosa, anorexia nervosa or compulsive eating.

Weight charts are designed to be guidelines (originally for life insurance purposes). But in the last few years it's been shown that being up to a stone over your highest weight is more healthy than being the same amount under your lowest guideline weight. And some people disprove these weight guidelines by looking better, and preferring to be, slightly fatter or thinner than the ideals. It's when you begin to drop under weight or go over a stone higher that you should start to be concerned. Being underweight is usually caused by illness, stress or anorexia – and leaves you vulnerable without enough nutritional reserves to call on for extra energy, illness or a trauma. Being over a stone overweight makes you vulnerable to cholesterol-related diseases, strain on the heart, varicose veins, foot problems and so on. See guidelines for body weight on p. 110.

These are the people who should be watching their diets for health. All the rest of us do it for fashion – and there's nothing wrong with that, so long as you don't take it *too* seriously.

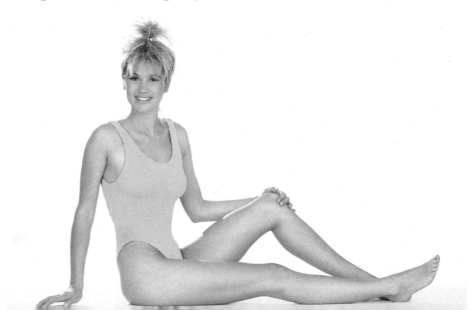

How to eat a healthy diet

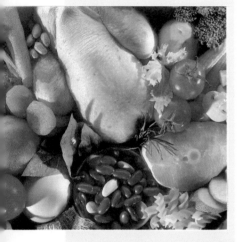

COLOUR-CODED DIET

VEGETARIAN AND VEGAN DIETS

This guide will give you all the nutrients you need to stay in top form. (But children up to 18, pregnant and breast-feeding women, those with heart disease or illnesses such as diabetes, have different requirements – please check with your doctor if you fall into any of these groups.) The weights in brackets are for those who'd like to lose around 2lb/1k a week – step up the amount of some of the portions in the Red section by half again if you find that you're losing more than this amount. Otherwise, use this plan, with sensible portions, for a balanced diet giving you all the nutrients you'll need. Obviously, you'll sometimes be confronted with foods not in the diet so try to work out which section they would come into and substitute them for foods already there (for example cake: Yellow section).

Normal eaters and slimmers. Each day eat three portions of the Green group; one portion from List A and one from List B of the Red group; two portions of the Brown group; one portion of the White and one portion of the Yellow group.

Slimmers. Use the bracketed cooked weights for a weight loss of around 2lb/1k a week. Men who are slimming need more calories and should step up Red group and Brown group portions by half again.

NB: Where there are no measurements, eat as much as you like within reason.

Normal eaters. Use this guide as a basis for eating a balanced diet – there is no need to weigh your portions.

NB: All weights refer to cooked weights of foods.

The vegetarian diet is, generally, a healthy one. But vegetarians, like everyone else, need to take care not to eat too much fat. They need to be careful about vitamin B_{12} which most people get from meat and eggs. Cheese and whole milk contain vitamin B_{12} but also quite a lot of fat, and therefore calories. Yeast extract also contains B_{12}. But, not surprisingly, nearly all vegetarian diets are high in

Green

different portions 3

Lettuce, broccoli, gooseberries, lemon, melon, lime, asparagus, Brussels sprouts, celery, cucumber, gherkins, marrow, onions, spinach, green pepper, seakale, artichokes, watercress, cauliflower, greens, cabbage, mustard and cress, courgette, herbs, Chinese leaves, chicory, beansprouts, (2oz/50g) peas or mange tout, (7oz/200g) green or runner beans, (5oz/150g) leeks, (1) apple, (1) pear, (3½oz/90g) grapes, (3oz/75g) greengages, (3½oz/90g) broad beans.

Brown

portions 2

(2½oz/70g) wholemeal bread, (7) wholemeal or bran crispbreads, (3) oatcakes, (5oz/150g) cooked wholemeal pasta, (5oz/150g) cooked brown rice, (7oz/200g) potatoes cooked with skins, (6oz/175g) cooked lentils, (1oz/25g) mixed nuts, (9oz/250g) baked beans, (9oz/250g) stewed prunes, (1oz/25g) wholemeal pastry, 1¾oz/45g) muesli or bran breakfast cereal, (7oz/200g) cooked haricot, butter or soya beans, mushrooms.

Yellow

1 portion from each section

(1oz/25g) hard cheese (Cheddar, Cheshire), (2oz/50g) Edam cheese, (2) eggs, (¾oz/20g) butter or margarine, (1oz/25g) double cream

(1oz/25g) sweetcorn, (6oz/175g) swede, (3oz/75g) parsnip, (6oz/175g) turnip, (1) large grapefruit, (2oz/50g) banana, (4fl.oz/125ml) unsweetened grapefruit juice.

White

portions 1

(5–6oz/150–175g) yoghurt, (½pint/300ml) skimmed milk, (¼pint/150ml) whole fat milk, (6oz/175g) white fish, (4oz/110g) cottage cheese.

Red

LIST A portions 1

(3oz/75g) salmon, (5oz/150g) mussels, (3oz/75g) drained tuna, (4½oz/125g) shrimps, (2oz/50g) herring, (4oz/110g) crab meat, (4oz/110g) fish roe, (4oz/110g) drained pilchard, (2oz/50g) mackerel, (3oz/75g) lean ham, (3oz/75g) lean lamb, (3oz/75g) lean pork, (4½oz/125g) skinned chicken, (3oz/75g) lean beef, (3oz/75g) duck, (3oz/75g) rabbit, (4oz/110g) turkey, (3oz/75g) offal (liver, heart or kidney, sweetbreads or brains), (1oz/25g) salami, (3) chipolata sausages, (6oz/175g) red kidney beans (well cooked).

LIST B portions 1

(3) tomatoes, (7fl.oz/200ml) tomato or unsweetened orange juice, (1) large orange, (12½oz/365g) watermelon, (10½oz/300g) strawberries, (9oz/250g) blackberries, (1lb3oz/500g) pumpkin, (7½oz/210g) passion fruit, (6oz/175g) cherries, (10oz/285g) apricots, (1) nectarine, (1×5oz/150g) large peach, (12oz/350g) plums, (9½oz/265g) blackcurrants, (10½oz/300g) raspberries, (15oz/420g) loganberries, redcurrants, rhubarb, (9½oz/265g) beetroot, cranberries, red pepper, red cabbage, radish, aubergine.

fibre which is fairly filling and, in moderation, good for health.

Vegans have an even more restricted diet. They don't eat any food of animal origin (for example cheese, milk, yoghurt, eggs). But provided they eat a wide variety of cereals, pulses, other vegetables, fruits, nuts and vitamin-fortified margarine, they are likely to get enough of all nutrients. Be sure to eat a good mixture at the same meal of pulses (peas, beans and lentils) and cereals (bread, pasta and rice) to get enough good quality protein.

General rules for vegetarian/vegan diets

Vegetarians should have skimmed or semi-skimmed milk, not full-cream or whole milk, to cut fat and calories. And go easy on hard and cream cheese. Even reduced-fat hard cheese, such as Cheddar, still contains quite a lot of fat. Vegans need to maintain calcium balance with soya and soya bean products such as tofu. Vitamin D is rarely found in plants but you can top up with vegan margarine; the law insists that all margarines are fortified with vitamins A and D. Outdoor light also helps the body make its own vitamin D – vegans should enjoy it whenever possible.

These diets are designed to lose you up to 2lb/1k a week on 1,100 calories; men need 350 more so should double portions for lunch. Each day have up to ½pt/300ml skimmed or semi-skimmed milk or soya milk, plain or in tea and coffee, in addition to the milk in the items listed.

Choose one breakfast, one lunch and one evening meal. But you can eat them any time of day you like. Vegan alternatives are in brackets. They should substitute these for the dairy products in each meal.

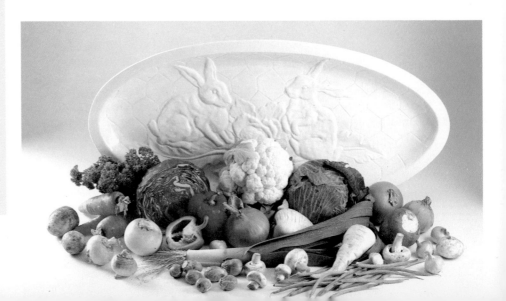

| **Breakfast** (200 Calories) | (1) ¾oz/20g Bran Flakes *or* 1oz/25g All-Bran *or* Puffed Wheat *or* 1 Weetabix with 1tbsp raisins or sultanas and ¼pt/150ml skimmed or semi-skimmed or soya milk.
(2) 1 slice wholemeal bread with very little butter or polyunsaturated margarine and 1tsp marmalade or honey.
(3) 1 slice wholemeal bread, 1 poached or boiled egg, 2 grilled tomatoes or ¼pt/150ml tomato juice. | 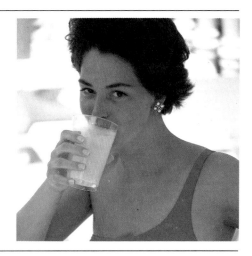 |

Lunch (350 Calories)

(1) 4oz/110g cottage cheese (or 2oz/50g chick pea spread), 2 crispbreads with very little butter or polyunsaturated margarine, tomato, cucumber and onion salad, 2 pieces fresh fruit.

(2) ½pt/300ml mixed vegetable or onion soup topped with 2tbsp grated Cheddar cheese (or containing potato, pulses, vegetables and 1oz/25g diced tofu), 1 slice wholemeal bread (+ 1 piece fresh fruit).

(3) Salad of 2oz/50g well-cooked and cooled or canned red kidney beans. 2oz/50g haricot beans or chick peas tossed in 1tbsp vinaigrette. Serve on lettuce and top with 1oz/25g bread cubes, toasted, 2 pieces fresh fruit.

(4) 2-egg omelette filled with 2tbsp mixed vegetables. Large portion sliced green beans, 2oz/50g peas. (Rice and bean salad made with 4oz/110g cooked brown rice, 1 stick sliced celery, ½oz/15g cashew or peanuts, 2oz/50g any cooked pulse, dash soy sauce and 1 tsp Hoi Sin Sauce. Tomato and cucumber salad. An apple or pear.)

(5) Sandwich made with 2 slices wholemeal bread and very little butter or polyunsaturated margarine, lettuce, tomato, 1tbsp grated hard cheese and 1tsp sweet pickle. (1 wholemeal pitta filled with 2tsp sweetcorn, chopped red pepper, any salad vegetable and dressing made by mixing 1tsp silken tofu, chopped parsley, little lemon juice, pinch of cumin and chopped onion.)

(6) 5oz/150g baked beans, 1 slice wholemeal toast, 2 grilled tomatoes, individual tub any low-fat fruit yoghurt and 1 piece fresh fruit. (Omit yoghurt: 6oz/175g fruit salad with purée of strawberries or raspberries.)

(7) Pasta salad: mix 3oz/75g cooked pasta shells, 2oz/50g cooked cut beans, 2oz/50g cooked haricot beans, slices from ½ cooked courgette, 2oz/50g poached button mushrooms, 1tbsp vinaigrette shaken well with 1tbsp tomato purée, 1 small banana.

Evening (420 Calories)

(1) 1 medium (7oz/200g) jacket potato: halve, scoop out, mash and mix with 1 tbsp sweetcorn, 1tbsp low-fat natural yoghurt (silken tofu), seasoning. Replace in potato shells. Top with 2tbsp grated Cheddar cheese (omit) and grill to brown and heat through. Mixed green salad with tomatoes, 1 piece fresh fruit. (Salad of cooked whole French beans, tomato, chopped marjoram, 4 olives and 1tbsp vinaigrette, 1 slice wholemeal bread.)

(2) ¼pt/150ml tomato or vegetable juice. Egg pasta: beat 1 egg with 1tbsp chopped parsley, nutmeg and seasoning. Mix with 6oz/175g cooked spaghetti and heat very gently until egg is just set. Top with 1 tbsp grated Parmesan cheese. 1 orange. (Pasta with aubergines: cut ½ small aubergine and 1 courgette in pieces. Cook in 3oz/75g canned chopped tomato with good pinch dried mixed herbs and a little chopped onion. Cook 2oz/50g pasta shapes, drain, add 2oz/50g diced tofu to aubergine mixture for the last 3 minutes of cooking. Stir pasta into vegetable mix, season.)

(3) Stuffed courgette: cook 1 large courgette whole until just tender. Drain and halve lengthways. Scoop out flesh, dice and mix with ½oz/15g flaked almonds, 2oz/50g cooked or canned chick peas, 1tbsp cooked chopped onion, 2tbsp white sauce (made with soya milk) and seasoning. Replace in courgette shells, top with 2tbsp grated Parmesan cheese (breadcrumbs) and grill to heat and brown. 2oz/50g piece French bread or 6oz/175g jacket baked potato.

(4) Bulgar wheat and vegetable curry: make a curry sauce in usual way but with as little oil as possible. Cook 2oz/50g bulgar wheat in stock for 10–15 minutes. Mix with diced cooked carrot, mushrooms, 1oz/25g haricot beans and 2oz/50g yoghurt (diced tofu). Serve with 2oz/50g raw weight boiled brown rice.

VITAMINS AND MINERALS

These are essential trace nutrients in food which are vital to the smooth running of the body. A healthy diet is one that supplies all you need. See under the Supplement section for special cases who may like to add more to their diets, but beware of taking more than the stated dose – it can do the body damage.

CRASH DIETS

Apart from being potentially dangerous, they don't work. You may have lost 6lb/2.7k in two days but, because this is mainly water, as soon as you start eating and drinking normally again, you'll put it

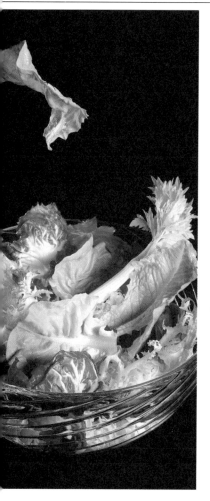

(5) Pasta ratatouille: cook together in 2tsp oil, 1 small diced courgette, ¼ small diced aubergine, 2tbsp chopped onion, 2 chopped canned tomatoes, pinch mixed herbs, seasoning; simmer until tender. Stir in 6oz/175g any cooked pasta shapes. 5oz/150g low-fat natural yoghurt topped with 1tsp honey. (Baked green pepper filled with cooked rice mixed with vegetables and 1oz/25g toasted nuts – flaked almonds or hazelnuts. Serve with tomato sauce flavoured with basil and a green vegetable purée such as Brussels sprouts.)

(6) Cauliflower and leek cheese: put 3oz/75g cooked pasta in an ovenproof dish. Add 4oz/110g cooked cauliflower and 1 cooked small diced leek, seasoning and 3tbsp white sauce (made with soya milk). Top with 2tbsp grated hard cheese (2tbsp breadcrumbs) and grill or bake to brown. Large portion green beans, 2 grilled or baked tomatoes.

(7) Spinach pancakes: make 2 thin pancakes (with tofu instead of eggs). Cook a little chopped onion in 1tsp oil. Add 10oz/275g frozen spinach, seasoning, pinch of nutmeg and 2 chopped canned tomatoes. Boil to evaporate water. Divide between pancakes, roll up and top with 2tbsp white sauce (made with soya milk) and 2tbsp grated hard cheese. Green salad (salad of lettuce, cucumber, spring onions, 1tbsp vinaigrette and chopped fresh herbs), 1 baked apple filled with 1tbsp raisins or sultanas.

Chick pea spread

8oz/225g cooked or canned chick peas, drained
1oz/25g crunchy peanut butter
1oz/25g tahini
3tbsp lemon juice
salt and pepper

Put all ingredients in a blender and blend until fairly smooth. A few pieces of peanut to add texture. Makes about 11oz/300g. Calories per oz/25g: 55.

back on. Meanwhile you're depriving your body of valuable nutrients that it needs to function properly. The average woman needs around 1,500 calories a day and will lose weight sensibly and surely on 1,100 calories (men on 1,500). Any less than this should be considered a crash diet. Certain vitamins, proteins and carbohydrates need regular topping up to keep your body healthy and your energy level high. When we deprive ourselves of food the first things to be affected are the parts that our ingenious system considers to be superfluous – nails, teeth, hair and skin condition. Our nervous system gets into gear to fight for the vital missing food, causing tension and bad temper. Instinct and a cleverly designed warning system evolved over millions of years come into play and let us know all is not well. Don't crash diet – it may allow you to get into the dress you want to wear for that special occasion, but you won't look or feel so good in it and can do yourself long-term damage.

FAD DIETS

These include anything that hinges on a particular food or eating pattern that you wouldn't normally eat or follow. They are usually named after places or the way they're structured. And unless you are prepared to alter your lifestyle drastically enough to accommodate a peculiar or anti-social eating programme, these diets are extremely difficult to follow. Usually, people begin to crave the foods that are 'banned' or wish to eat at times that they're not 'supposed' to. Although some of them aren't actually harmful, these diets will take over your life, make losing weight more of an ordeal than it should be and are usually impossible to follow for any length of time. Some people may have success with them but then have the added trial of learning to eat normally again afterwards without putting weight back on . . . It's easier to learn the lesson from the beginning with a varied and balanced eating programme which will fit in, long term, with your lifestyle.

ANOREXIA NERVOSA AND BULIMIA NERVOSA

Both are psychological disorders affecting the appetite. Anorectics starve themselves but still appear fat to their own distorted view. Bulimics binge food; then purge themselves through vomiting or laxatives. Both disorders need professional help but unfortunately a symptom of these illnesses is an inability to recognise the condition and a determination to keep the related behaviour secret. While an anorectic becomes extremely thin and will, at the worst, starve to death, bulimics can be of normal weight and carry on the bizarre eating pattern for years. Seek help from your GP – many of whom now recognise these illnesses – if you think that you, or someone close to you, is suffering. And bear in mind that these illnesses affect men too.

SLIMMING CLUBS

These can be fun for those who enjoy slimming in company. They are a source of advice and support. While some take themselves very seriously and the competitive element is high, the larger national slimming clubs can provide good specialist information and support for those with diet-related diseases (diabetes, heart disease) from their years of experience. It is wise, however, to visit your doctor if you've recently been ill to ask her/him to vet a new diet, if you're not sure that it comes from a qualified nutritionalist who is an expert in your particular problem. If there isn't a slimming club near you and you feel it would help you to lose unwanted weight, why not start one?

SLIMMING ACCESSORIES

Low calorie or low fat substitutes. Substitute foods include everything from saccharin and sugar-free foods to low calorie pre-packed meals and skimmed milk. They can be useful in place of higher calorie foods; that is in moderation and as part of a balanced diet. Additives like preservatives and colouring in processed foods (as opposed to raw ingredients which you cook yourself) can have adverse effects on some people and you should seek a doctor's advice if you think these may be affecting you. For others, the occasional pre-packed slimming meal or using sweeteners, instead of sugar, in up to six cups of tea or coffee a day will do no harm – so long as it's balanced with natural food (particularly fruit and vegetables). Some pre-packed foods are carefully balanced to make sure they contain good quantities of the nutrients you need on a low food intake. Others warn on the pack that they should only be used in conjunction with a nutritionally balanced diet. Better and less expensive is to learn to swap certain foods for healthier alternatives – high-fibre bread (with wholemeal or added bran), natural fruit instead of sugary puddings, yoghurt instead of cream, purées instead of fatty or creamy sauces, raw fruit or vegetables (which contain more goodness than when they're tinned, frozen or cooked – except kidney beans which are dangerous when eaten undercooked). These are the real slimming substitutes.

Slimming aids. Some slimming aids are meal substitutes, and increasingly, nutritionalists believe that these are not good for you. Not only are they very low calorie, which could leave you nutritionally deficient, especially if you have a medical condition affecting your diet (pregnancy or diabetes), but as they're also often in liquid form, the lack of roughage can upset smooth running of the digestive track, resulting in constipation. These products do not educate you to eat properly. The idea of a balanced, low calorie diet is to lose you weight while allowing you to eat the kinds of widely available foods that you would normally eat. When you reach your goal weight, you can keep it stable by gradually stepping up portions, occasionally adding treats such as biscuits, chocolate or alcohol.

Fillers. Methylcellulose is sold in chewy cubes or added to foods to expand with liquid in the stomach, making you feel full – and it's not a good idea for those who wish to get used to eating less. High-fibre bran and roughage products fill you up but mostly aren't absorbed into the system, so help digestion without adding many calories. Bran is fine if used in a controlled manner – and the best way is combined with foods such as cereals, bread and so on. Too much can cause diarrhoea and discomfort.

Diuretics help rid you of retained water. Synthetic diuretics can cause symptoms such as nausea and dizziness while depleting the body of minerals. Those who suffer from mild oedema (bloating) should try instead the natural diuretics, in moderation: herbal teas, caffeine (as in coffee and tea), lettuce, cucumber, celery, broccoli, oranges, radishes and, finally, water itself are all diuretics and help to expel spare water from the body. Restricting salt intake helps, too.

Appetite suppressant drugs. Many of these potentially harmful and habit forming drugs are now either off the market completely or 'restricted'. They are still sometimes given to the very obese under medically controlled supervision. Anyone who is physically fit and just needs a boost to the willpower to lose a couple of stone should avoid them and find other ways of restricting calories.

Massage. See section in Chapter 10.

WHAT'S IN FOOD?

Protein. Essential to all known life and part of every living cell in the body: needed for growth, repair and can be used for energy. Meat, fish, offal, rice, pasta, pulse vegetables, nuts, cheese, eggs, milk and bread are rich in protein.

Fat. The most concentrated of all energy foods (protein and carbohydrates are the others but they contain less than half the energy of fat). You need certain types of fats from foods to keep you healthy as well as to supply energy. But fat is easily stored in the body if you eat too much. (Fat accounts for 28 per cent of the

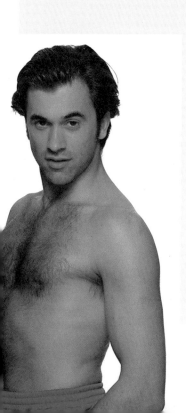

average body weight in women.) Saturated fats are usually non-liquid at room temperature, as found in butter, meat, hard margarine, palm oil and coconut oil. Too much can lead to cholesterol build-up in the blood and arteries leading to heart and vascular problems. Cholesterol also occurs naturally in food (shellfish, eggs, liver and other offal are high in it) but is mainly made in our bodies from saturated fats that we eat. More unsaturated fats are usually liquid (olive oil and nuts). Polyunsaturated fats, mostly from vegetable oils are also liquid and have the added advantage of reducing the level of cholesterol in the blood.

Carbohydrates are needed for heat and energy. Starch, sucrose (table sugar) and glucose come under the carbohydrate heading and are found in potatoes, pasta, rice, bread and fruit – dried fruit is a good healthy source when you feel energy levels are low.

Water. The most essential nutrient of all and second only to oxygen for survival. We can survive weeks without food but only a few days without water. The body consists of up to 60 per cent or on average 9 gallons/40 litres of water – which is constantly being used in every chemical process taking place in the body to keep us alive and well, then flushing away waste matter through the digestive and urinary track. Although you get water from foods, it's wise to make sure you drink at least four pints/two litres a day (more in hot weather).

Calories. Kilocalories or joules are the units of energy in foods and are essential for survival, but in *excess* they accumulate as fat in the body. All fats are high in calories. Carbohydrates (sugars and starches) and proteins also contain calories. Water, vitamins and minerals contain no calories, whereas fibre contains only a very small amount. Expend more calories than you take in and you lose weight. Joules are the international equivalent of calories. One calorie equals 4.2 joules. A kilojoule (KJ) is 1,000 joules.

Fibre or roughage. High fibre or roughage foods add bulk and give a satisfied feeling while supplying the body with less calories (or nutrients). Plant-based roughage includes fibre foods such as bran or wholemeal cereals (brown rice or flour, for instance, where the outer covering of the seed isn't removed by refining). Fruit and vegetables contain fibre; beans, pulses, peas, lentils, sweetcorn and baked beans are a good source. As high-fibre foods run through your system without being completely digested, they aid the smooth running of the digestive track. But don't overdo it, since recent reports claim that many people find too much fibre causes digestive problems.

SUPPLEMENTS

Over the past few years, many of us have tried to supplement the nutrients in our diets. Manufacturers of pills packed with vitamins, minerals, fish oils, plant essences, bee produce (royal jelly or honey and so on) have claimed all sorts of beneficial effects from taking them. The fact is that, if you're healthy and eating a varied and balanced diet, you don't need to supplement it. However, there's evidence to suggest that some people may benefit from supplementing so long as they don't exceed the proper dose (and aren't allergic to the colouring or preservatives). Here are those who might benefit from supplements:

Pregnant and breast-feeding women, those on the Pill or taking hormone treatment: Vit C (natural sources: citrus fruits, strawberries, blackcurrants, tomatoes, green and leafy vegetables, potatoes).
Folic acid (dark green leafy vegetables, offal, nuts, wheatgerm).
Vit E (some natural sources: nuts, seeds, wheatgerm, margarine, butter, cod liver oil).
Vit D (fatty fish, eggs, butter, margarine, or manufactured in the body in response to sunshine).
Vit B_1 (meat, liver, poultry, seeds and nuts, dairy products, green vegetables).
Vit B_2/riboflavin (liver, nuts, kidney, dairy milk).
Vit B_6 (bananas, chicken, avocado, tomatoes).
Calcium and phosphorus (fish, dairy products, dark green vegetables), iron (offal, oranges, green veg).

Night workers, the infirm or housebound (who don't get outside), the darker skinned and those whose customs decree covering their bodies outside: Vit D (some natural sources for non-vegans: milk, butter, Pacific salmon, mackerel).

Vegetarians and vegans: Vit D, Vit B_2/riboflavin, Vit B_{12} (kelp, peanuts, bananas, fish).

The elderly: calcium, phosphorus, folic acid, pantothenic acid (wholegrain breads and cereals, nuts, egg yolks, offal and chicken).

Smokers: Vit A (liver, carrots, green veg), Vit C, Vit B_1, Vit E.

Drinkers: Vit C, Vit B_1, B_{12}.

If on drugs (especially antibiotics): Vit C and B group vitamins.
Women suffering from pre-menstrual tension: Vit B$_6$, magnesium, evening primrose oil, zinc.
Those with strenuous jobs: sodium and chlorine (salt).
Those who have recently been ill: multi-vitamins and minerals.

TO PRESERVE THE NUTRIENTS IN YOUR FOODS:

Try to eat them as fresh as possible. Don't leave them in sunlight or a warm kitchen. Unlike poultry, you should try to eat vegetables and fruit with the skin on, where possible. When cooking, cut fruit and vegetables into as big chunks as possible and cook for minimum time and in minimum amount of water. Don't use copper pots or pans. Avoid bicarbonate to keep greens, bright green – it depletes Vitamin C content.

TIPS TO A HEALTHIER DIET

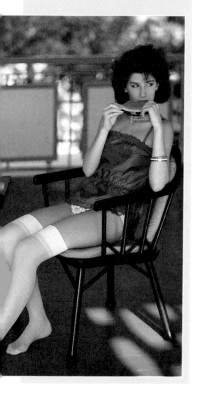

Eat as many different foods as possible at each meal.

Eat raw foods when possible.

Read the labels on pre-packed food and avoid those with added sugar and too many colourings or preservatives (these won't do most people any harm within reason). Ingredients are listed in descending order of weight, so the highest weight appears at the top of the list.

Go for bulk – wholemeal, wheatgerm or bran in bread, pasta, flour, cereals, etc.

Take the skin off poultry but leave it on fruit, vegetables, nuts and rice (brown) where possible.

Go for lean meat and cut the fat off. Opt for fish or skinned chicken more than red meat.

Grill or bake rather than fry – drain fat (for instance, from mince or a roast) before going on to prepare a meal.

Use minimum amounts of fat in cooking. Play up herbs and purées in recipes, instead of white sauces.

Swop to skimmed or semi-skimmed milk. Use polyunsaturated margarines instead of butter where possible – you soon get used to the different taste.

Moisten and line sandwiches with vegetable extract, lettuce or cottage cheese instead of fat.

Use yoghurt instead of cream or custard on puddings.

Put chopped herbs on vegetables instead of butter; spices on fruit instead of sugar. Choosing ripe fruit will avoid the need to balance the acidity with sugar.

Drink more water – especially before and with meals – to fill you up and help digestion.

Use fruit instead of sugar to sweeten cereals.

Cut down on alcohol and when you drink go for 'dry' instead of 'sweet' – the drier the beverage the less sugar it contains.

If you can, eat a good breakfast – you need nutrition after the long night's fast.

GUIDELINES FOR BODY WEIGHT

WOMEN

Height	Acceptable Range				
ft ins	st lb	st lb	cm	k	k
4 10	6 8–	8 7	147	42	54
4 11	6 10–	8 10	150	43	55
5 0	6 12–	8 13	152	44	57
5 1	7 1–	9 2	155	45	58
5 2	7 4–	9 5	157	46	59
5 3	7 7–	9 8	160	48	61
5 4	7 10–	9 12	163	49	63
5 5	7 13–	10 2	165	50	65
5 6	8 2–	10 6	168	52	66
5 7	8 6–	10 10	170	54	68
5 8	8 10–	11	173	55	70
5 9	9 –	11 4	175	57	72
5 10	9 4–	11 9	178	59	74
5 11	9 8–	12	180	61	76
6 0	9 12–	12 5	183	63	79

MEN

Height	Acceptable Range				
ft ins	st lb	st lb	cm	k	k
5 2	8 –	10 1	157	51	64
5 3	8 3–	10 4	160	52	65
5 4	8 6–	10 8	163	54	67
5 5	8 9–	10 12	165	55	69
5 6	8 12–	11 2	168	56	71
5 7	9 2–	11 7	170	58	74
5 8	9 6–	11 12	173	60	75
5 9	9 10–	12 2	175	62	77
5 10	10 –	12 6	178	64	79
5 11	10 4–	12 11	180	65	81
6 0	10 8–	13 2	183	67	84
6 1	10 12–	13 7	185	69	86
6 2	11 2–	13 12	188	71	88
6 3	11 6–	14 3	190	73	90
6 4	11 10–	14 8	193	75	93

CHAPTER 7

The Body Beautiful

An attractive body not only needs to be in good shape but should also show off soft, smooth, silky skin while smelling sweet. Daily bathing – whether by shower or bath – and checking perspiration along with superfluous hair, if you wish, will keep you nice to know and allow you to stay that way throughout a long or busy day. And no discussion on keeping your body looking beautiful would be complete without mention of how to sunbathe safely. For despite our increasing awareness of how the sun can damage our skins and the rising incidence of skin cancer in this country, we still think of a golden suntan as a symbol of beauty and luxury.

Baths and showers

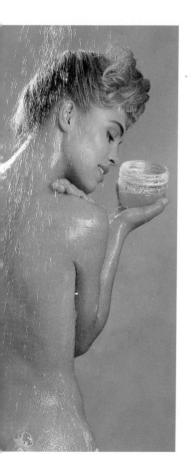

Bathing regularly is a recent occupation – and beauty treatment. We haven't always been so scrupulous about hygiene in Britain. For even though the ancient Romans left us public bathing buildings after their occupation of this country, it wasn't until the last century that baths were considered important enough to be installed in some houses. It was as recently as during Queen Victoria's reign that the noble and rich caught on to bathing for hygiene. During our grandparents' time, warm baths were thought effeminate for men; cold ones were considered masculine and proper!

Now 95 per cent of homes have a bath or shower and 65 per cent of women take a bath every day or every other day (compared to 45 per cent of men). Recently showers have gained in popularity. This is mainly because they are more cost effective, using less water and therefore less heat. The beauty advantages of showers are that they are less dehydrating to skin; soaking in water for a long time can make skin soggy and remove too much natural oil. Showers allow dirty water to drain away, while supplying a constant spray of clean water. They are also speedier and more invigorating, save time and wake you up in the morning or after a strenuous exercise session. Cleansing shower products (usually gels or mousses) can often be used for washing hair, too, and usually come with a handy hook for easier use; making losing or slipping on the soap a thing of the past!

However, if you like to relax and warm up in a bath, the therapeutic effects are well known. Sometimes used for calming down mentally disturbed patients, a steamy soak can have the same effect on you after a long day. You can treat bathtime as a haven away from the family by locking yourself in the bathroom. So make sure your bathroom is a place in which to relax and meditate. Soft lights, soothing music, something interesting to read and perhaps a glass of wine will all help the day's cares and worries dissolve with the dirt. Adding something smelly to the water completes the atmosphere. You should emerge more relaxed in mind and body. Warm water helps ease tired aching muscles but make sure you don't make it too hot. Around 94–98°F/34–36°C is about right. And avoid dryness and waterlogged skin by only submerging yourself for up to 15 minutes.

A DASH OF SOMETHING SCENTED?

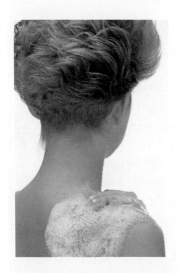

Different smells in your bath water can have all sorts of different effects on you. There are essential oils and preparations for calming, soothing, healing and energising. But remember to avoid perfumed products if you're prone to allergies or thrush. Instead, clean skin with unperfumed mild soaps or cleansing bars.

Soaps will clean skin but can be rather harsh for drier skins. Cleansing bars which look like soap but match your skin's pH acid/alkali balance may be a better bet if you suffer from skin complaints. Cleansing bars don't lather so much as soap but clean just as effectively.

Bath salts, cubes or crystals aim to soften harder water and allow lathering products to work better. They are not cleansing in themselves but will give you fragranced, and sometimes coloured, water.

Bubble baths are usually not moisturising (check the pack). So although these contain detergent for cleansing, as well as a booster for bubbles and perfume, they can be rather drying to the skin. Their advantage is that they don't leave a ring round the tub.

Moisturising bath oils and lotions don't cleanse but add droplets of perfumed oil throughout, or on top of, the water. When you emerge, these cling to your skin, leaving a fine layer to seal in moisture.

IN THE BATH

During your bath, the heat will help widen skin pores, so it is an ideal time to put on a deep cleansing face pack or apply conditioner to your hair to allow it to sink in more effectively. This is also the time to gently attack the build-up of stubborn fat you want to get rid of. Use a special massaging glove or pummel carefully with your clenched fists. Dispel hard skin around ankles, heels, toes, knees and elbows while it's softer with a loofah, pumice stone or the exfoliating creams which contain small granules to wear away skin. Softened skin is more vulnerable and can be damaged easily by too rough treatment so avoid over-enthusiasm.

AFTER YOUR BATH

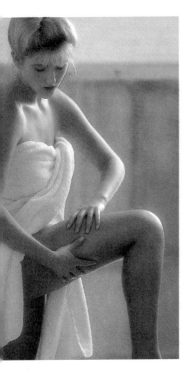

Ideally you should dry off naturally. If this isn't practical, put on a fluffy absorbent bath robe or pat yourself dry with a towel. Vigorous rubbing with a towel will damage sensitive skin and remove the benefits of a moisturising bath oil. This is also the time to gently push back softened cuticles or cut softened nails, if they need it. Apply deodorant and talc to the areas where wetness occurs and, before drying off completely, apply a luxurious layer of body lotion to seal in the moisture.

Whirlpool baths (or Jacuzzis) aim to massage your body with jets of water as you soak. But be careful; too much jet pressure or getting too close to the source of an underwater spray can cause bruising. Make your own whirlpool bath by giving yourself an underwater massage with a hand-held shower.

Turkish baths use steam to help rid the body of waste matter through sweating. This application of heat, with massage, aims to deep cleanse and relax you.

Mud baths. Mud is said to have antiseptic properties and helps exfoliation. So bathing in it is believed to help healing and skin health.

Salt rubs. Coarse sea salt acts as an exfoliation for top dead skin. It is rubbed on to damp skin then rinsed off to expose newer, softer skin.

Saunas are not advised for those with high blood pressure or heart disease. These wood cabins are heated with burning coals to reach very high temperatures. As you perspire, water is added to the coals for humidity and you then emerge to plunge into an icy pool or take a cold shower. How long you remain in the heat and how many times you repeat the process, varies with individuals.

Steam cabinets enclose all your body, except head, and subject it to steam treatment to cleanse and lose you weight. (But water weight loss, like this, is quickly replaced again when you drink.)

Cooling down

Sweating is the way we cool down and excrete waste products. On average you sweat around four pints/two litres a day but this can go up dramatically in hot weather or during strenuous activity – when you need to be sure to replace lost liquid by drinking more. Some people naturally sweat more. Heat, spicy foods, embarrassment, feeling sexy and hormonal changes (such as puberty, pre-menstruation or during the menopause) can all lead to increased perspiration. We've probably all come across someone who *doesn't* keep their personal hygiene in check. Here's how you can make sure it isn't *you*.

It's not actually perspiration that smells but sweat mixed with skin bacteria which has gone stale. So make sure you bath or shower regularly using a good cleansing soap, shower or bath product. Also make sure you clean your clothes regularly (change underwear, tights, socks or stockings every day), allow shoes, coats and jackets to 'rest' between wearings.

Now some methods to keep perspiration to a minimum:

Choose cotton underwear and clothes made from natural fabrics to help skin 'breathe'. The looser fitting, the better. Avoid synthetics.

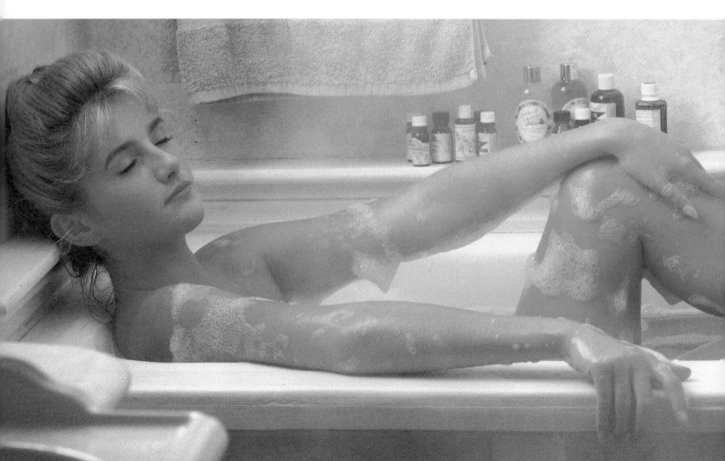

Lukewarm water for showers or baths is more cooling and stops skin reacting to extreme heat or cold.

Opt for stockings instead of tights or go without either and fake tan legs in the summer for a cooler feel. Keep feet cool and dry by wearing open sandals.

A water spray will refresh and cool you down.

Cut down on spicy foods, alcohol, caffeine, and avoid stress which can cause more sweating. Drink plenty of liquids to avoid dehydration.

When possible, run cold water over your wrists or your feet; in hot weather, it will cool you down.

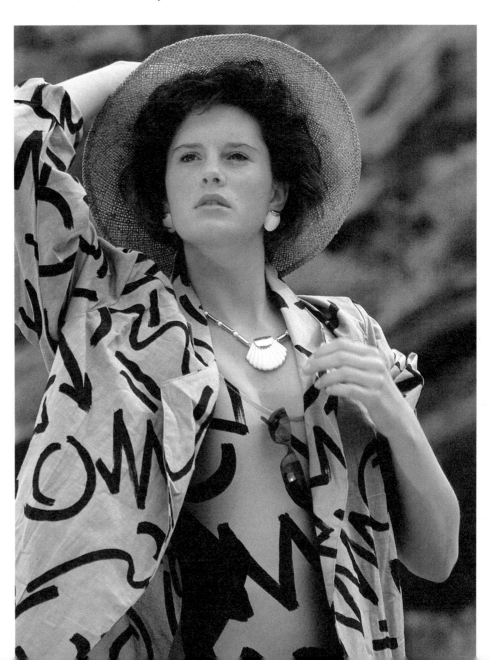

Feet: Wear leather rather than synthetic shoes. Wash feet twice a day and dust toes and inside shoes with medicated foot powder.

Keep your temper! Studies in America show that hot weather can mean hot headedness. It's best to count to 100.

Deodorants and anti-perspirants are the best preventive measures for staying nice to know. Deodorants disguise smell in the same way as a perfume and have an antiseptic or bactericide ingredient to inhibit bacteria. Anti-perspirants also help stop wetness by constricting or plugging pores to prevent perspiration escaping and contain covering perfume and bactericide. But no anti-perspirant will stop sweat completely.

Where should you keep cool? The eccrine sweat glands over most of the body produce perspiration consisting mainly of water, which is less likely to smell. Important areas for odour are where the apocrine sweat glands are found – underarms, genital region, around nipples and naval. The sweat produced here contains a higher percentage of fatty matter and salts which, when trapped for long periods, decompose skin bacteria and cause odour. Apocrine glands develop at puberty; this is why children don't suffer from body odour.

How to get the best from your deodorant/anti-perspirant. Apply it to clean dry underarm skin after bathing. Roll-ons, sticks and creams are more effective than spray-ons; though sprays are more hygienic for family use. Removing underarm hair means anti-perspirant is in closer contact with skin after application, but don't apply it for a few hours after defuzzing and never on 'nicked' or sore skin. One application in the morning after washing should help keep you smelling sweet throughout the day.

Allergy prone skins prefer unperfumed brands.

Those with excess perspiration should try heavy-duty anti-perspirants – check at your chemist. If these don't solve the problem, see your GP.

Where else? Most dermatologists recommend avoiding the delicate skin around genitals, but body sprays can freshen the rest of you. Special strong foot and shoe anti-perspirants can prevent feet from becoming anti-social.

Hyperidrosis is excessive perspiration caused by being overweight, or by an over-active nervous system. See your doctor if you feel it is hindering day-to-day life.

Bromidrosis is a medical symptom of some conditions such as kidney disease in which sweat has an unpleasant smell.

Defuzzing

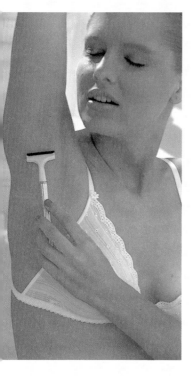

Unlike in some European countries, British women still spend considerable time and money on trying to remove what they consider surplus hair. Why? Presumably the idea dates back to the days of poor hygiene and hair nits when a smoother skin meant better cleanliness.

However there are some practical reasons for removing, say, leg or underarm hair. It's cooler in summer; it stops interference with a tan, and most of the British still perceive bodily hair as unattractive.

Hair all over our body (yes, most women have it everywhere though not as heavily as the hair which arrives at puberty in underarm, pubic and leg regions) served originally to keep us warm. As clothes now do this job, anthropologists believe that in a few thousand years we'll be hair free – and that includes our head hair disappearing, too!

But until then, if one of your biggest beauty bores is ridding yourself of unwanted hair, here's how you can do it:

Underarm
Can be creamed, shaved or waxed.

Depilatory creams dissolve hair to just under the skin surface in 10 to 20 minutes; then you simply wash it away. The disadvantage is that the chemical smell (calcium thioglycolate) is detectable, however heavily disguised by the manufacturer's scent; although many are trying to resolve this. You may need to resort to another method with stronger hair. Try a patch test 24 hours before using a new depilatory for the first time (obviously somewhere that you'd like to be hair-free!) as the allergy rate to hair removal creams is quite high.

Shaving armpits is quick and easy but you may find you've a five o'clock underarm shadow anything from a few hours to a day later. Cheap disposable razors mean you needn't worry about cleaning blades or rust. But be careful not to nick delicate skin here as it's not the easiest place to see; only those with a steady hand should use wet razors, perhaps with a special ladies' shaving mousse. Others may like to try one of the battery-operated, lady-shave razors. You can use most of them wet or dry but check the pack first to make sure that they're waterproof.

Waxing underarm hair can be painful as it's a delicate area.

Legs

Can be shaved, creamed or waxed.

Waxing is ideal for larger expanses and less delicate skin, and it will allow you to stay hair free for three to five weeks depending on your rate of hair growth. First experience of waxing can be a bit of a shock. It's like pulling off a plaster, so it stings. But hairs get weaker, the more you wax. Take an aspirin beforehand, if you have a low pain threshold. You can have hair waxed in a salon or you could try one of the at-home kits. These are either ready-waxed strips or kits of heatable tubs of wax (or a wax-filled roll-on container), with material strips. The strips are pressed over the area (after wax is applied in a thin layer with the kit) and then pulled off against the direction of hair growth bringing hairs with it. Hot wax is applied in a layer, allowed to set and pulled off when solid.

Both waxing and shaving remove the top dead layer of skin. So a cooling moisture lotion will help stop stinging. You should be careful not to expose unprotected skin to sun for 12 hours afterwards.

Bikini line hair is usually stronger and situated inside upper thighs making legs look less attractive in swimsuits. Waxing is probably the best method here as shaving leaves stubble and creams aren't so easy to control (you have to sit still for 10 to 20 minutes). In a salon, a therapist will wax away hairs to your swimsuit line (take it with you to make sure).

Facial hair may be creamed, waxed, tweezed or bleached. Apply a warm flannel then tweeze the odd one, pulling in the direction of growth, but avoid hairs in moles or covering large areas. Creams made especially for faces should be patch tested first and remember to read instructions carefully. The same applies to bleach. Or you may consider electrolysis.

Odd straggly hairs on back, stomach, around nipples and so on are ideal candidates for *electrolysis*, which is the only permanent hair removal method. It *must* be carried out by an experienced operator with a certificate from the British Association of Electrolysis, 18 Stokes End, Haddenham, Bucks HP17 8DX or a diploma from The Institute of Electrolysis, 251 Seymour Grove, Manchester M16 0DS (enclose an SAE for a list of qualified operators). If you're not sure, the bigger department stores are the best bet. In electrolysis a fine needle is put into the hair follicle and an electric current runs down it to kill the root. You will need several sessions (depending on strength of hair) before the root is permanently destroyed. And you may experience some discomfort while it's being done (opinions vary from 'it tickles' to 'Chinese torture'). If you can't bear the thought, pluck out stray hairs.

A recent addition to the removal method which does not claim to be permanent is *tweezer epilation* in which the tweezers are attached to each hair and current applied.

Excess hair can be caused by hormonal imbalances, often at menopause, but it can also be hereditary. Sudden growth of excess hair may also be a symptom of hormonal problems. Hormonal drug treatment prescribed by your doctor is only suitable for some people as it affects the whole body. Visit your GP for further information.

Suntanning

A golden tan makes eyes and teeth look whiter while boosting morale and vitamin D in the body. But the dangers to health may make you think it's not worth the risk. If you do decide to go for gold, do it in the safest possible way.

The suntan process starts when ultraviolet (UV) light from the sun activates melanin production deep in the skin. UV light is broken down into three types: UVA, UVB, UVC. Don't worry about UVC as this is mainly broken up outside the earth's atmosphere and rarely reaches us. UVB is the burning ray which starts skin going red in seconds after first exposure. UVA (the principal one used in sunbeds) is the long ray which doesn't burn easily but goes deep into the skin and is now said by dermatologists to give the more far-reaching damage associated with sunbathing (such as premature ageing, sagging skin, skin deformities and cancers like melanoma – a tumour of brown pigment cells).

Melanin is a brown pigment produced by the body in response to UVA and UVB to help protect us from light damage. This pigment gives you your tan. Some of us naturally have more in our skins and therefore more natural protection from the sun. Basically, the darker you are the less likely you are to burn and damage your skin. Black people have most natural melanin so have less chance of damage, while albinos are least protected without sunscreen.

Dermatologists say that longterm bouts of sunbathing will age you quicker (as much as 20 years more at 40 years old) and increase the risk of developing skin cancers and melanoma (very pale skins are twice as likely to succumb). All types of skin cancer are increasing and it is now the most common form of cancer in the Western world. This is a direct result of suntanning. You must weigh up the risks and decide if you think sunbathing is worthwhile.

The safest way to tan is by opting for a fake or self-tan product to give the appearance of suntan. Or if you are a sun worshipper, gen up on all the facts. First assess your skin colouring. There are five types and men have the same as women:

Fairest of them all. Always burns, rarely tans. Often redheads, with freckles, light eyebrows and green or pale blue eyes.

Fair and fine. Always burns, sometimes tans. Blondes or brunettes with light coloured skins prone to allergy or irritation.

Normal. Always tans, sometimes burns. May have blue or brown eyes but never look ultra-pale in the winter.

Dark. Always tans, rarely burns. Most often brunettes with dark brown eyes and sallow complexions.

'Black' skins. Afro-Caribbean complexions very rarely burn. After you've worked out your skin type, other influences may affect tanning. Check this list: the Pill, pregnancy, taking hormone replacement drugs, some antibiotics, tranquillisers and sleeping tablets can cause deeper pigmentation patches (chloasma). Check with your doctor before sunbathing. Perfume (and don't forget scent in soaps, make-up and deodorants) can cause photosensitivity with allergic reactions or uneven pigmentation. And remember that depilatory creams contain scent; shaving and waxing remove the top layer of skin making it more sensitive – so make sure you defuzz at least 12 hours before exposure.

Newly exposed skins (babies and small children, people with healed burns, grazes or scars) aren't so hardened to the melanin producing process and are more likely to burn, so initially need extra strong protection.

Gauge your surroundings. The nearer to the sun you are (on top of a hill, near the Equator) the more intense the sun's rays. Likewise, the time of day. In Britain it's around midday, in other countries it may vary anywhere between 11 am to 3 pm. And the weather can be deceptive – you *can* burn through light cloud or haze. You may think you're safe in the shade or under water without protection. Think again! The sun's rays are reflected upwards (up to 80 per cent of them on snow, a lesser amount on sand and paving stones) and they can reach down to three feet under water.

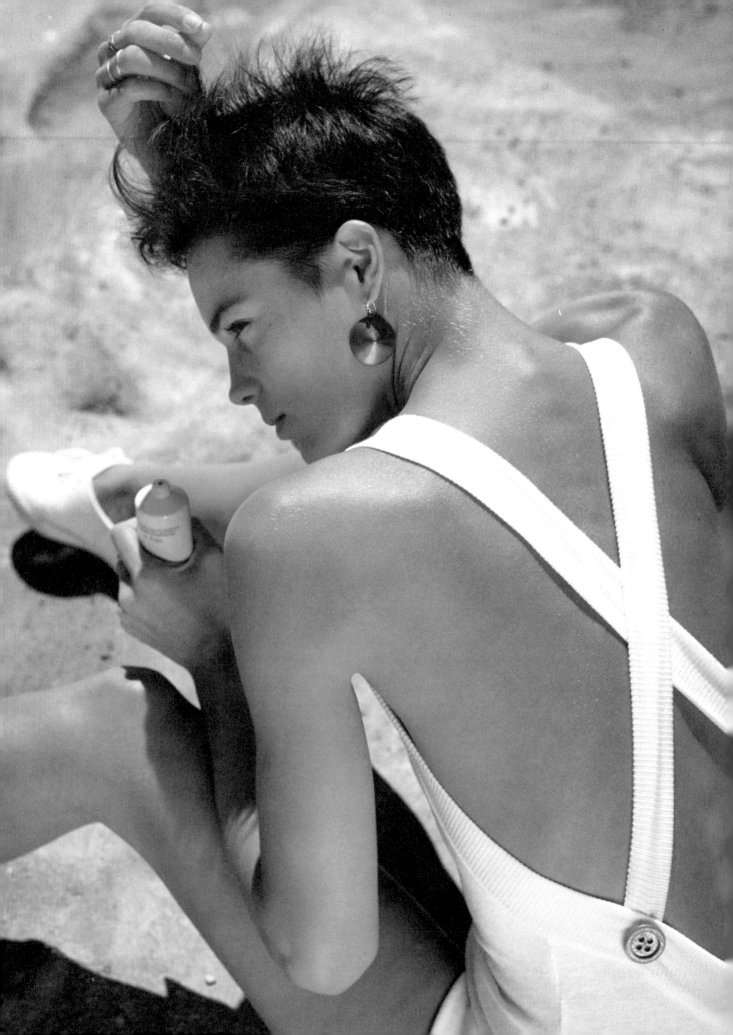

PROTECTION

Melanin produced by sunbathing should take three to four days to reach the skin's surface and give a bit of colour. Any sooner and you're likely to peel. Although the skin needs to get a little flushed to start the boost of pigmentation formation, this should go after 12 hours. If it doesn't, you've burnt and are likely to start peeling straight away. The way to control your sunbathing is by the use of sunscreens containing Sun Protection Factors (SPF).

What are SPFs? The number of a Sun Protection Factor represents the amount of time you can stay in the sun without burning compared to having no protection at all. For instance, if you've normal or fair skin with a slight tan and can take 15 minutes in the sun before you start stinging, a SPF of 2 will give you half an hour (15 minutes $\times$ 2 = 30 minutes). SPF 6 will allow you one and a half hours of burn-free bronzing (15 minutes $\times$ 6 = 90 minutes). You can also use SPFs to vary your time in the sun. Supposing you're on holiday and want to spend four hours on the beach. You're already quite tanned and can take up to half an hour of mid-morning sunlight without burning; an SPF 8 will allow you those four hours' protection, whereas if you've only a lunch hour to top up your tan, an SPF 2 is all you need.

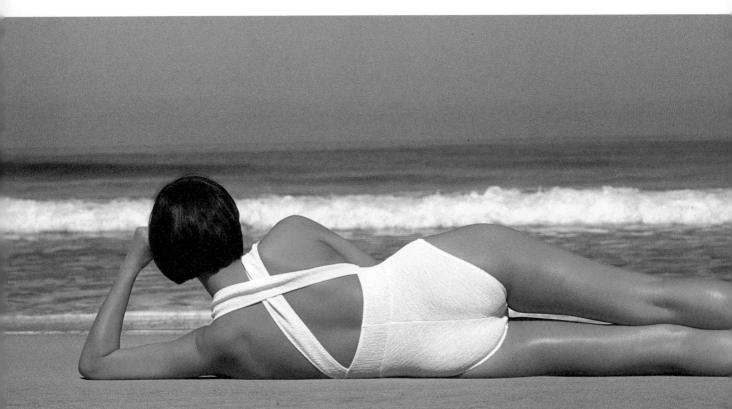

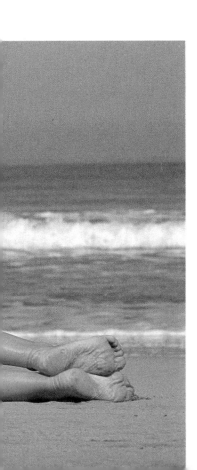

A word of warning: SPFs vary from country to country. Here in Britain they're usually to the American, Swiss or German standards. American SPFs tend to provide lower protection (in other words, the on-pack SPF numbers are higher) than European ones. So until they are standardised, err on the side of caution, opting for a higher number than you think you need if you're not sure – whether you buy a sunscreen product here or abroad.

And buy the SPF you need for your skin type:

Fairest of them all. Should not attempt to tan as you will always burn. Products calling themselves sunblocks vary enormously in their protection factors, from SPF 8, which should be reapplied every 40 minutes for maximum protection, to SPF 22 which will last a couple of hours. Most are around SPF 10 to 15 and should be reapplied after one hour and 15 minutes.

Fair and fine skins should start off with 10 minutes of unprotected exposure going up by five minutes a day for maximum safety. You can multiply these figures by the SPF sunscreen you're using – and go on to a sunblock if you've used up allotted time. Allergy-prone skin should use an unperfumed range, but do a patch test first to be sure. Well done those suncare manufacturers who've included UVA, as well as the usual UVB filters, in their sunscreens. Those with fair, fine skins are most at risk from the dangers of UV light.

Normal. Start with 15 minutes of unprotected exposure going up by 10 minutes a day. Multiply these figures by the SPF you're using to give you safe tanning with sunscreen. Waterbabies should seek out water resistant products but check the instructions thoroughly to see how long protection lasts in the water. Normal skins might also like to use a tinted sunscreen to take the glare off whiter-than-pale skin while they brown. Some fake tans have a low degree of protection.

Dark and black skins. Dark skins which hardly ever burn are rare but obviously the darker your skin, the less likely you are to burn. But even black skins may burn in prolonged, intense sunlight and darker skins do get dehydrated. Try a moisturised sunscreen, on the basis that you'll probably be able to stand around half an hour in the sun unprotected on first exposure.

Make sure you apply sunscreen in a cool place to dry, clean skin which has been moisturised at least an hour beforehand. Damp skin, from perspiration or moisturiser, will dilute the protection. Read the instructions carefully to see when you need to re-apply and use liberally to give you maximum protection at all times. Don't towel dry after a dip – you'll rub off even water resistant screens.

Melanin boosters. These tan accelerators aim to push melanin production in the skin into gear faster on exposure to the sun. Usually they are applied up to three days before sunbathing. They act as a photosensitising agent to the skin and have a high incidence of allergy and/or uneven pigmentation. Dermatologists report greater vulnerability to skin cancer but as yet there's no conclusive proof.

Tanning pills. Apart from being dangerous to health, these can turn you orange all over (including on the palms of your hands). They have been reported to cause nausea and, more seriously, can cause deposits in the kidneys and eyes.

Sunbeds are growing in popularity and are installed in most health or beauty clubs. Originally, they were considered safe as they emit minimum amounts of burning rays (UVB) and maximum tanning rays (UVA). Now dermatologists have found that the UVA tanning rays do deeper damage at the level where new skin cells are formed. Sunbeds are more dangerous than sunshine as there are so few burning rays to start skin stinging and warn you that you're damaging your skin. If you do decide to use a sunbed, always wear goggles to protect your eyes and make sure that the sunbed has been cleaned with a disinfectant product before you lie down. Do not use a sunbed every week.

SKIN AFTER SUN

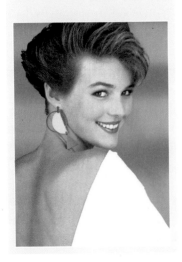

When you're overdone the sunbathing you need to apply a good soothing after-sun lotion. These are specially formulated to soothe and cool down sore, stinging, red skin. They'll also give some moisture protection to help prevent the skin dehydrating and peeling so easily. After-sun lotions which say they're cooling usually include an ingredient which has a slight numbing effect on the skin to make soreness less painful. But if you're really sore, try calamine lotion or a first aid spray from the chemist, as these have a stronger anaesthetic effect. If you've sunburnt skin, take a shower (it's less dehydrating) or bath (if you must) in tepid water – too hot or cold will aggravate skin and make you feel even more sore.

If you also have a headache and dizziness, you may have slight sunstroke. The cure is rest and liquids. Lie down in a darkened, well ventilated room and drink plenty of fruit juice or mineral water until symptoms pass. If you still feel ill after 12 hours or start to develop large blisters, contact a doctor immediately. *Never* expose red, blistering or peeling skin to the sun again. And be sure to use a high protection sunscreen after you've peeled and you're trying to tan new, pale skin.

FAKE TANNING

Whatever the weather or your skin type, you can go beautifully brown in the comfort of your own home in a matter of hours. Fake, or self-tans as they're sometimes called, have nothing to do with the sun but work by reacting chemically with the skin or coating it with make-up.

A *long-lasting tan* takes three to six hours to develop and lasts for up to a week. In 1959, a colourless aftershave lotion in America claimed to produce gradual tanning within six hours of application. The active ingredient which did this was isolated as dihydroxyacetone (DHA). DHA reacts with amino acids in the protein, at the upper layers of skin, to form dark-coloured pigment after a few hours of application. This is the base of the most semi-permanent type of self or fake tan preparations on the market today, and they are now available in cream, lotions or foams from chemists and major department stores.

When to fake it:

You're worried about the sun's effect on your skin. You like being brown but don't wish to risk premature ageing or skin cancer. You're photosensitive to sunlight (an allergic reaction caused by antibiotics, tranquillisers or sleeping pills) or it brings you out in brown patches (chloasma – sometimes caused by the Pill or pregnancy).

It's warm enough to go bare legged but you don't want to expose pure white legs. Leg make-up was first used during the war – it was called Stocking Cream when nylons were hard to get – but modern self tans don't streak in the rain and can last for up to a week.

You find sunbathing boring and it leaves you red instead of golden brown.

You've already got a stunning, golden glow except for two lily white bikini strap marks.

Your existing tan is beginning to pale and is in need of a boost.

You go on your annual search for the sun for two weeks and it rains non-stop.

You're stuck in rainy Britain for the summer!

Application: Self-tanning products vary in strength and from user to user. A good golden glow on one person may become a streaky orange flush on another. It all depends on skin type (natural shade and condition), application and product. But here are some useful guidelines to follow to ensure the best results.

Dry skins with rough patches are going to show up fake tan more on the drier parts as they have a higher degree of absorption. Hence the problems some people encounter with tide lines round feet, knees and elbows. Skin is thicker in these places too, and so again able to absorb more, giving a darker concentration of colour. The answer is to smooth and moisturise the skin at least two hours before application. If you have areas of skin with blemishes or rough patches where more than one moisturising session is needed – fake tans aren't for you until the patches disappear.

Greasy or perspiring skins dilute and help streak the product. Tone oily skin on face with an alcohol based toner before application, and make sure you're cool and dry before and, for at least an hour, after application.

Natural colour of skin matters, too. Sallow or already tanned skin can stand stronger or more applications as any discrepancies in coverage won't show through so easily.

Already self-tanned skin should be treated in the same way as dry skin before you proceed. The gentle use of a body buffer or buffing products will slough off patches of old fake tan, leaving an unblemished surface on which to re-apply. Fake tan can build up in patches in already tanned or dry areas and although it might not show with one application could become all too visible with two.

Products vary in strengths and the other ingredients in a fake tan might affect eventual colour, too (some contain more alcohol or moisturiser).

Most mistakes are made by not rubbing in fake tan enough. As it is initially invisible, be sure to apply evenly and rub in thoroughly. Greasier skins can take foams as they don't contain so much moisturiser but these may sink in too quickly and give uneven colour on dry patches.

It's wise to test a fake colour for your skin type and shade on an area which won't show such as the top of your leg. Do this at least six hours before you want to see the results. Then decide whether to be more sparing or generous in your application. In general, fake tan should sink in easily after a minute, although foam ones always take less time. If you're still rubbing it in after this time, you've applied too much.

Some self-tans are blended with sunscreen agents and walnut extract or henna so that you have immediate sun protection from the dyes and a sunscreen effect with the pigment formed later by DHA. Read the instructions very carefully to find out exactly what your fake tan will do.

If your product states that it will protect you from the sun on
application and pigment doesn't appear for a few hours, it means it
also contains a sunscreen (though this may only be low). All DHA
fake tans will give some degree of protection from the sun by their
colour once they are developed on the skin.

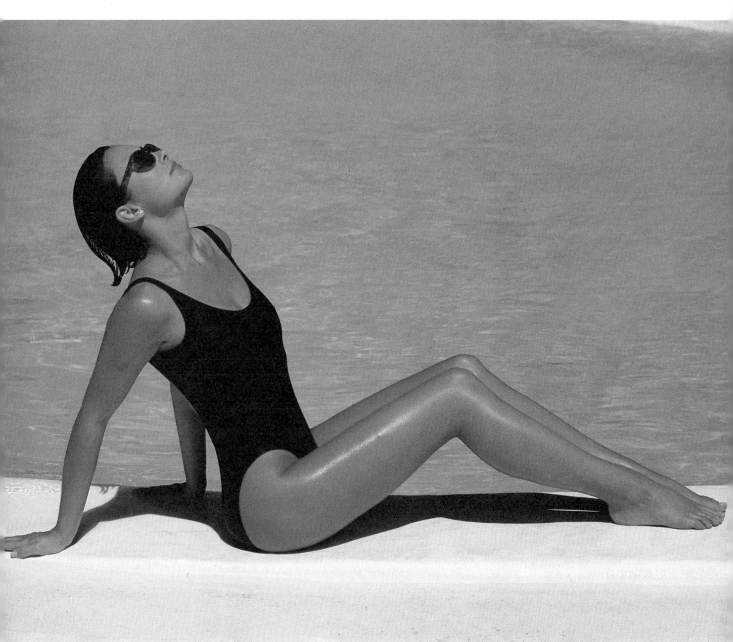

Remember to:

Wash palms of hands thoroughly after application or you'll end up with them stained.

Fade off application around base of fingers and toes, soles of feet, armpits, inside arms, hairline – anywhere you don't normally tan. Do this in stroking movements towards those areas. Do the same around elbows, where fake tan tends to gather and concentrate in colour.

Don't let skin, with fake tan applied, contact clothes or bedding for at least an hour after application.

Fake tan may darken grey or light hair, wool or nylon.

Colour should gradually fade over one week. Re-apply after six hours for a deeper shade or when you think skin needs a top up.

Wash-off tan tints give an instant, temporary colour. They are usually strong pigments in an alcohol or gel base and you need to have well moisturised, smooth skin and apply with care. Wash-off tans come in coloured lotions, gels, powders and tinted moisturisers. Some are water resistant, others wash off like ordinary make-up with soap or cleanser and water to avoid streaking. Tinted moisturisers containing a sunscreen are ideal for faces.

CHAPTER 8

Forgotten Assets

Even though our hands, bottoms, legs and feet support and work hard for us every day, getting more wear and tear than other parts of the body, we tend to forget them when it comes to keeping them healthy and beautiful. Because of their supporting roles, they're also more likely to suffer from dry, rough skin or problems associated with friction or pressure. Yet by looking after your forgotten assets, they'll not only be a beauty bonus but will also serve you better.

Handy hints

The Chinese started reading hands as far back as 5000 BC. And the psychiatrist Carl Jung is said to have been interested in the art of expressing character through hands. 'Hands, whose shape and functioning are so intimately connected with the psychic, might prove revealing,' he wrote.

Did you know, for instance, that broader fingers convey open mindedness, tolerance and generosity, or that square-shaped fingers mean you're rational and ordered? But apart from expressing our personalities, hands do plenty of work so they need help to stay in good shape. Hands reveal age – and there is little you can do to make them look younger when they're wrinkled (though there's nothing to stop you putting facial anti-wrinkle treatments on them if you can afford the quantity needed). Better is to make sure you keep them moisturised. Once a week, use a heavy cream and be prepared to let it sink in for about 20 minutes. Make it a rule to use handcream every day and also to apply hand or body lotion on hands before putting on rubber gloves to immerse them in water. The heat helps the moisture to sink in – a bit like a deep conditioning treatment.

Care for your hands with a thorough *manicure* at least every two weeks (condition nails at least every week). The manicure should take from 15 minutes to half an hour. Remove all dead polish and wash immediately to get rid of the drying residue. Keep the

fingertips soaking in warm water for a few minutes to soften cuticles
and nails. Now trim nails with a pair of sharp scissors made for the
job. Push back cuticles gently with the curved end of an orange
stick or with your thumbnail – but don't push too hard as you may
damage the delicate skin where the new nail is forming and cause
dents or white specks on the nail. If you're prone to hangnails, use a

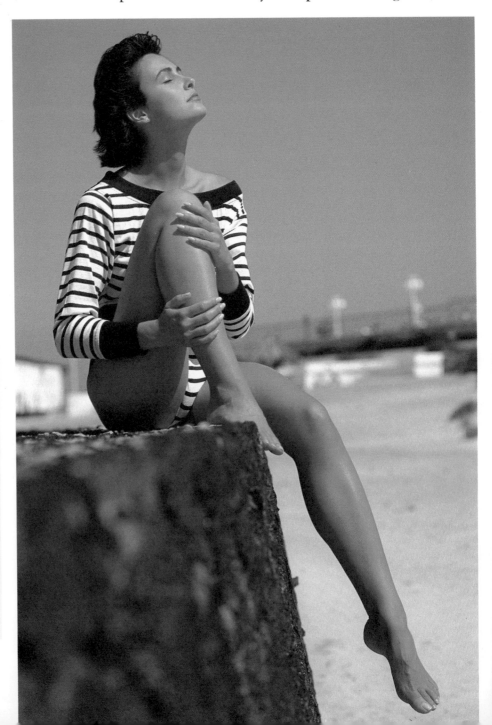

nail clipper, carefully, on longer skin tags. Now file nails with an emery board (metal files can be too harsh and cause splitting). File in one direction (side to centre) rather than in a scrubbing motion, creating a gentle curve; filing too far down at sides can cause hangnails. The most practical length for fingernails is from level with tip of finger to ⅛″/3mm over. Use a good conditioning cuticle cream and give yourself a hand massage while it sinks in. Apply a generous amount of softening cream and smooth it over hands up to wrists. Then, using the thumb and forefinger of the other hand, work from each fingertip to wrist in stroking movements. Then apply more cream and work from wrist to fingertips on each hand. Buffing your nails gives them a healthy shine and speeds up circulation, making them glow with health; you can put polish on top if you wish.

To strengthen weak nails, try a nail hardener. Mend broken or split nails with a mender kit, available from chemists.

False tips come in a kit with glue and different shaped nails. Just stick them on and paint over with polish. Remove with varnish remover. The latest cosmetic treatment from America, available from some beauticians here, is silk wrapping. Nail extensions are fixed on, shaped, then fine silk strips are applied to the whole nail. Filing and buffing help blend them on and give an illusion of natural glowing nails. There is no need to apply polish over them unless you wish.

Exercise hands by pretending to play the piano or by typing. Knitting also keeps fingers supple. Get circulation going by stretching arms out straight and making fists then stretching out fingers as far as possible. Repeat 15 times.

Make stubby fingers look longer by wearing delicate rings and thick chunky bracelets. Paint a single stripe of bright polish down the centre of nails (leaving sides unpolished). Or leave nails clear so as not to draw attention to them.

Polish. A recent innovation is a spillproof varnish pen that gives you nail colour and dries twice as fast as ordinary polish but hasn't yet got the shine and consistency of bottle polishes. A base coat is always a good idea before applying polish, to prevent the nail being stained by deep colours. Match nail colour to your lipstick, jewellery, even eye make-up. Aim to cover nail by painting in two strokes from cuticle to tip, and allow to dry thoroughly before applying another coat. Keep down chips by using a strengthening top coat which seals the nail and gives extra hard cover.

Feet first

As they're furthest away from our head, they're usually last in our beauty thoughts. But neglect your feet and they'll soon let you know. Tired aching feet affect your whole body and certainly your facial expression – so it's worth looking after them. There are 26 bones in *each* foot so with all the attached tendons and muscles there's plenty to go wrong and keep chiropodists in business. Being overweight and wearing badly fitting shoes are the worst things we can do to them. Feet 'spread' as we get older, even though we stop growing at around 18; so make sure you're still taking the right shoe size. Healthy feet should be allowed to breathe and exercise as often as possible. Try walking around barefoot at home (or in winter with just cotton socks). Changing shoes, boots and sandal shapes along with varying heel height will work different sets of muscles and keep feet in shape.

Care for your feet with a regular *pedicure* at least every two weeks. Remove all old polish and treat yourself to a footbath with a special foot balm or moisturising bath lotion in warm water (bottom of the bath, washing up bowl or bidet are ideal for this). Or try a foot spa, which is available at chemists and a bit like a whirlpool bath for feet. When skin is soft, buff off dry flaky skin with a pumice stone. Buff especially around the big toe, side of foot and heel. Now pat dry and trim toenails straight across. Best length is to the end of the toe; file jagged edges (but not corners as this could lead to ingrown toenails) and gently push back cuticles with thumb. Now rub in some nail conditioning cream.

A special foot lotion or cream is formulated to help cool them down and keep feet smooth and fresh. Massage lotion on in stroking movements from the end of the arch near heel to top near big toe. Now hold each toe between finger and thumb and press from the base upwards. When you get to toe top bend it back for 10 seconds, then forwards (as far as it'll go without hurting). Another good exercise for feet that can be done anywhere (watching TV, at a desk, alone in the dentist's waiting room) is, when sitting down, to lift one leg straight out and point big toe forwards. Now make circles in the air with your big toe, making sure you just rotate the ankle and keep the leg straight. Go clockwise 20 times then anti-clockwise. Repeat with other foot. This aids circulation and can help swollen, tired or cold legs and feet.

Glamorise feet with some beautifully coloured toenails. After

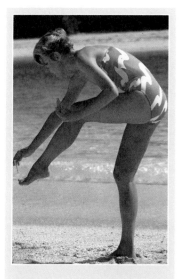

conditioner has sunk in (give it half an hour), apply a clear base coat. If toes are close together, try cotton wool between them to keep them apart while painting. Good shaped feet look stunning with a layer or two of bright coral, brilliant red or orange polish for summer – and try some gold for special effect in the evenings. Others should stick to pastel shades such as peach or shell pink.

Best cure for swollen feet (and on the pressurised cabin of a plane they can swell up to a size larger – remember this when choosing shoes for travelling) is to put them up higher than your hips after arriving at your destination. Another tip for aiding circulation to feet when you've been standing for a long time is the Queen's own, and an old guardsman trick – to slowly rock backwards and forwards from ball to heel. It really works!

Sweaty feet are more likely to suffer from fungal infections. Try an anti-perspirant for feet and dust between toes with a good foot powder, too. Otherwise carry some freshen-up tissues with you while travelling and blot feet for freshness when you find a convenient place. Avoid wearing trainers or synthetic shoes too often. Serious excess foot perspiration is a medical problem – go and see your doctor.

FOOT PROBLEMS:

Athlete's Foot. A fungal infection easily caught and characterised by itchy, flaky red patches between toes. Treat with anti-fungal sprays or powders to dry them out. Keep feet dry, wash them often and don't go barefoot or share towels with others.

Verruca. A type of contagious wart usually on the soles of feet. Consult your chiropodist who may treat with an exfoliant solution available from the chemist. Keep covered with plaster until treatment finishes.

Corns/Calluses. Hard patches of skin which have built up under friction or pressure (usually caused by the wrong walking posture or badly fitting shoes). Remove minor ones by sloughing with a pumice. A chiropodist can remove more stubborn patches but they'll come back unless you deal with the original cause.

Bunions. Inflamed large joints of foot caused by injury or badly fitting shoes and not so easily cured (usually only by an operation). See your chiropodist.

Ingrown toenails require an operation if they're painful. See a chiropodist in the first instance.

To find a good chiropodist ask at your GP's surgery, local library or town hall. Or contact The Society of Chiropodists, 53 Welbeck Street, London, W1M 7HE tel: 01 486 3381, who will be able to put you in touch with a trained one in your area.

Foot healing. Reflexology is an ancient type of foot massage popular again today. It claims to diagnose and cure ills in the body by special pressure on the foot. Reflexologists believe that there are energy channels running throughout the body, terminating at your hands and feet. Clearing these channels through pressure at the right point on the foot aids health in the corresponding part of the body.

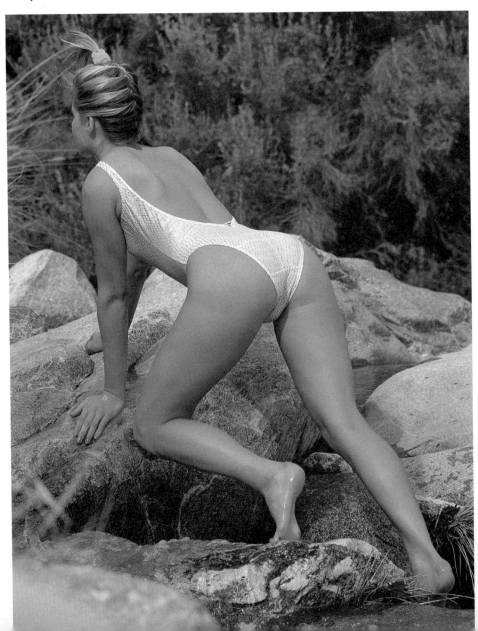

Legging it

Your bottom, thighs and legs provide a soft padding to sit on; animals who don't sit down on this part of their anatomy have not evolved the same kind of spare cushioning flesh around their hind quarters. Fat here also provides a nutritional store after pregnancy for breast-feeding mothers. Fatter hips and thighs go in and out of fashion – just think of Renoir's large-hipped ladies compared to today's big-busted, slim-hipped fashionable look. With recent slimmer styles, high-cut swimsuits and mini skirts, no one wants to show sagging, dimpled flesh on their bottoms and hips, but as we don't see our own rear ends often these areas tend to be neglected.

Unfortunately the Great British Pear Shape is hereditary and part of our heritage! If you've inherited it, you will only lose weight off this area through dieting (see Chapter 6). But exercise can firm you up as you trim off inches and keep you smooth and well shaped.

Try these exercises every day for 15 minutes:

Lie straight out on your side, head supported by your hand, one leg on top of the other. Lift top leg up straight, pointing toe at ceiling. Swing in an arc down to ground in front of you (remembering not to bend knee) and then up and back behind you. Do this 10 times, turn over and repeat on the other side.

Now get up and, turning sideways with back straight and arms out straight at sides, one holding on to the back of a chair or ledge at waist level, stand on tip toe and then bend knees as slowly as you can until your bottom touches your heels. Slowly again, come up to a standing position. Do this 10 times.

Now swing outside leg out high to your side, without bending knee and with foot pointed back straight. Try to make large circles in the air with your toe. Do this five times, then bring leg down and repeat with other leg.

Lastly, try to walk across the floor on your bottom, with legs and hands out in front of you!

Anytime, anywhere clench your buttocks together, hold for three seconds and release. Repeat as often as possible.

A flattering illusion for hips is to make your waist smaller so that you appear more curvy. Try touching toes, using a hula hoop or gently swinging your body from side to side from the waist to trim it.

Dimply skin. Cellulite is the name for puckered, orange-peel looking skin which is hard to shift (see Chapter 6). Avoid jeans or

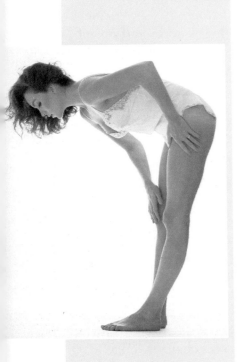

underwear that are too tight – these restrict lymphatic drainage in these areas and so help keep a waterlogged layer under the skin. Exercise helps and so does massaging with a knobbled massage glove.

Stretch marks on thighs – as on stomach – after weight loss or pregnancy can't be dispelled completely. A good softening lotion helps keep skin moisturised and smooth but won't prevent them, although they do fade with time. Disguise them with a fake tan.

Varicose veins occur when a valve in a vein stops working properly; blood flow is impeded and blood collects in pools, causing swelling veins. Left untreated they can cause ulcers and eventually thrombosis. Varicose veins begin with aching, tired, itchy legs. Although the tendency to suffer is inherited, they're aggravated by being overweight, by constipation, sitting with legs under you, prolonged standing, weak leg muscles, pregnancy and an unbalanced diet. Your doctor can give you prescriptive tablets, if you seek treatment for varicose veins early. These reduce inflammation and help blood flow more smoothly. Shorter veins can be injected to seal the vein. Longer veins can be surgically removed (involving a two- to four-day hospital stay). Exercise to build leg muscles helps prevent varicose veins, and support tights (which now come in lightweight 15 denier) hold veins deeper in the leg and ease aching. Avoid knee socks, hold-up stockings or anything that impedes blood flow in legs. Never massage over varicose veins.

Pimply, spotty skin is a surface skin problem and can be cured in the same way as spots on your face. But it becomes more of a problem when legs are enclosed in tights and trousers all winter. Try to go barelegged when weather is warm or stick to stockings and high-cut briefs to allow thigh and bottom skin some fresh air. Treat spotty areas by thorough cleansing with a medicated face wash; then use a medicated gel.

Make legs look longer when you've shaped and smoothed them by wearing high cut swimsuits – they flatter legs and make them look longer. But don't forget to remove bikini line hair.

CHAPTER 9

In Good Health

There is nothing more important to you and those close to you than being in good health. You can change your looks (easily), your weight, your lifestyle, your job, your home. But strong teeth and bones, good vision, a clear head, a healthy pregnancy and freedom from worries like cancer can give you the basis of a good lifestyle, great looks and help you to achieve all your dreams. Cosmetic surgery concerns general wellbeing, too – appearance can affect your health and you need to be fit and well to undergo these operations. Here is not the place to go into ways of easing the more

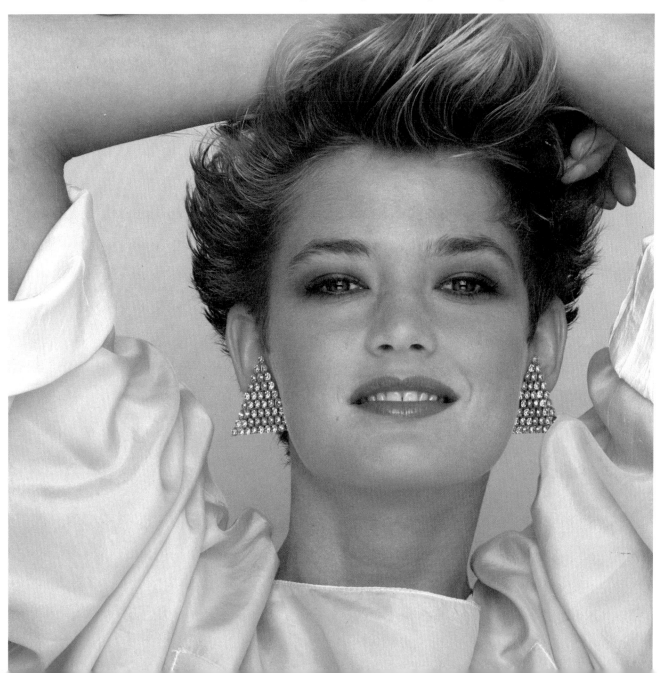

unfortunate, long term and disabling diseases such as multiple sclerosis, diabetes and cystic fibrosis which deserve a book each, but to show you how you can keep yourself and your family in sparkling form and prevent problems where none should be allowed to exist.

Teeth

A bright smile can make you appear more intelligent while bad breath is affecting the sex life of three out of ten couples (38 per cent suffer from it). How is that for an incentive to keep your mouth and teeth in tip top condition?

Bad breath is caused by bad teeth or gums, stomach complaints, eating spicy foods, drinking tea or coffee or smoking. Chewing parsley is said to help reduce it. Or try a fluoride mouthwash from your chemist.

Stained teeth can be caused by tobacco, coffee, red wine or strong food dyes. Also by rotting teeth or poor cleaning.

TEETH CARE

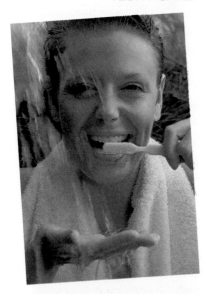

As many as nine out of ten adults in Britain are reported to be suffering from gum disease. This can lead to loose teeth, abscesses and bone damage. But the good news is that by really looking after your teeth you can prevent damage and keep all your pearlies well into old age. That means watching what you eat, brushing with a good fluoride toothpaste (fluoride has been proved to help strengthen enamel against bacterial damage) and twice daily flossing to stop plaque attacking teeth.

What is plaque? A near invisible, jelly-like substance that sticks to teeth. Mature plaque, whether white or stained, is nine-tenths composed of harmful bacteria, which inflame gums and decompose sugar into acid, leading to tooth decay.

Tartar is hardened plaque on the tooth surface, either above or below the gum. It has a rough surface, which makes new plaque cling more easily.

DAMAGE THAT CAN'T BE HELPED

You can't help being born with a bad bite (either badly sited teeth or a misformed jaw) or having teeth damaged through accident. Nor, say the experts, can you help having weak teeth or bacteria which are predisposed to forming harmful plaque. Hormonal (Pill, pregnancy) or health changes can affect gums and the possibility of tooth decay. But there is no need to lose a tooth for every baby you have, if you take extra special care with dental hygiene during and after pregnancy, although some antibiotics taken during certain stages of pregnancy are thought to have longlasting harmful effects which may discolour your baby's teeth.

PREVENTION TECHNIQUES

In a 1983 survey, 48 per cent of five year olds in England and Wales were found to have some tooth decay. And this figure, although decreasing over recent years, went up to 93 per cent for 15 year olds.

So what can you do to stop harm to children's teeth? One answer is to *time* tooth brushing. As over two minutes of thorough brushing is recommended, try a timer to make sure the full time is taken. Children should be encouraged to use dental floss from an early age to establish good habits. Besides, first (or deciduous) teeth set the site for second, permanent teeth; so early extractions can cause lasting malformation. Find a dentist who encourages children to visit – perhaps with video games or toothbrush clubs available in the surgery.

Pits and fissures on teeth (the bumps and ridges where bacteria can't be easily brushed away) can be sealed with a type of tough transparent plastic coat soon after a permanent tooth is through. And although dentists can't guarantee that sealing will stop decay completely, this pain-free treatment, taking about 10 minutes, has been proved to help prevent it. Some community dental clinics will provide fissure sealing free.

Another survey has shown that the more frequently you eat sugary foods (rather than the quantity) determines how much teeth decay. So if you can't persuade children to give up sweet foods completely, allow them only at *one* time of the day, after a meal and preferably an hour or two before brushing teeth. Encourage snacks of fruit or raw vegetables or give another non-edible treat instead. Be extra scrupulous about brushing after taking syrup cough mixtures. Adults and children should brush and floss teeth at least twice a day. A dental hygienist (at most dental surgeries) will show you how to do this efficiently, without damage to teeth. And it's now believed that a water jet, which plugs into a shaving socket, may help your gums.

You can't do much about naturally yellow teeth, but teeth with surface enamel stains caused by coffee, red wine or smoking may benefit from a 'polishing' toothpaste. Ask your hygienist how frequently to use these, as they can wear away the valuable enamel covering your teeth. Latest dental research is into combating harmful bacteria in your mouth to prevent them causing decay. Unfortunately, these treatments may not be widely available for some years.

WHAT TO DO ABOUT BAD TEETH

As you become older you may become 'long in the tooth'. Gums recede with age to expose more tooth. The first ones are usually the eye teeth, at the corners of the mouth, which are subject to more wear than others. Gums should not bleed when you brush teeth; if they do, the chances are that you've already got some gum disease. The first stage is *gingivitis*, where the soft tissue of the gum becomes red, swollen and sometimes bleeds. *Periodontitis* is the later stage; in this the supporting bone is affected, too.

Gum disease starts with plaque attacking the area where gums and teeth meet and forming a pocket between them at the gum. If allowed to remain over a number of years, it will deepen, attack roots and bone and probably form an abscess. The tooth will become loose, but by this time you're sure to have noticed that something is wrong – although abscesses aren't always painful.

Here are some dental techniques that can help correct bad or disfigured teeth:

Orthodontics is both a means of straightening crossed, crowded or irregular teeth by braces (either fixed or removable) and a term for surgery on the jaw. How often, and how long, the braces are worn depends on the individual problem. Sometimes teeth are extracted to make more room in an overcrowded mouth. Most often orthodontic procedures are applied to children whose second teeth have just fully formed (around 10–12 years). But sometimes teeth incline out or sideways with age, and so orthodontics can be performed at any age. Ask your dentist about charges under the NHS.

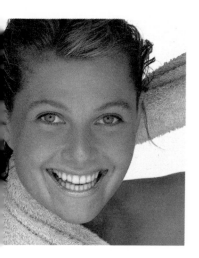

Fillings. As back teeth have to withstand the force of chewing, they are traditionally filled with an extra strong, silver-coloured mixture of silver, tin, copper and mercury called amalgam. The latest finding is a strong, tooth-coloured composite material which can withstand the pressure of eating and is more able to stick to the tooth, so may require less drilling before filling. This is not available at NHS costs for back teeth (only front), so if you'd like natural coloured fillings in your back teeth, ask your dentist for prices.

Root canal work. When decay reaches the nerve in the middle of the tooth, it may die. The tube inside the tooth is filled with bacteria and dead tissue, which will eventually cause an abscess. Root canal work cleans and then seals this tube, so there is no live tissue inside and disease has been removed to prevent further damage.

Veneering or bonding can only be used on healthy front teeth to repair a broken tooth, fill gappy teeth or give stained or discoloured teeth a natural shade. After teeth are cleaned and polished, then prepared with a weak acid solution to produce a rough surface for adhesion, a clear plastic coat is painted on to the enamel surface. Then tooth-coloured material is placed on to the tooth; it is set by light and smoothed to the right shape. The dentist may use a ready made, laminated veneer stuck to the tooth by similar method. Bonded teeth may stain or damage more easily than natural teeth and so sometimes need to be repaired or re-covered after a few years. Your dentist may be able to obtain NHS approval for non-cosmetic cases.

Filing should not be done just for appearance. But it will provide a better bite if one tooth sticks out or is chipped. Causes of why the tooth is sticking out should be investigated first. Costs for filing should be included in the basic NHS charge.

Crowning should only be considered when teeth aren't completely healthy, as it shortens the life of a healthy tooth and encourages gum recession. Crowning consists of the tooth being filed to a peg, then careful measurements and impressions are taken to make the cap. A temporary crown is put on until the permanent one is ready (usually a week). Success depends on the skill of the dentist and technician making the crown. A good crown may, with care, last for a lifetime, although it's not unusual to have one replacement. Ask your dentist for maximum NHS charges for a porcelain crown or how much a gold one will cost.

Bridging is done when one or two teeth are missing (or have to be taken out) and false teeth are attached to either one, or both, of the remaining teeth on each side of the gap. Bridges aren't designed to be removed. Usually the stable adjacent teeth are cut down to pegs and the whole structure fixed over both the gap and the pegs – so you need strong supporting teeth. Cost depends on the work involved and it will be more expensive than a partial denture. As each unit is costly and you'll usually need at least three of them (two for the supporting teeth), you will probably pay at least the maximum NHS charge.

Partial or full dentures. Removable partial dentures on a plastic or metal plate can clip onto existing teeth to fill the gaps. Extracting all your teeth for full dentures should be the dentist's last resort, and only done if too many teeth have already come out or you have progressive, untreatable gum disease. False teeth are made of plastic, or sometimes porcelain, with a plastic or metal base. After all natural teeth have been extracted impressions and careful measurements are taken to ensure dentures fit neatly over the gum without rubbing or moving when you talk or eat. There's usually one 'fitting' before finished dentures are ready. Comfort of the denture depends on the skill of the dentist and technician. As gums shrink, dentures may need relining. Have them checked at least every five years. There is a maximum NHS charge for traditional plastic or metal plate dentures.

Implants. This is when metal pegs are inserted into the bone of the jaw to support the dentures. They arc not suitable for most gums and are not generally available as dentists rarely recommend implants unless other dental techniques are not possible.

Transplants. In this a healthy tooth is transplanted into a more obvious space. They have been successful but there is a risk of rejection and you'll need to go to a specialist private dentist.

GOING TO THE DENTIST

Choosing a new dentist isn't easy. All dentists providing NHS care are listed at the Family Practitioner Committee in your area (in Scotland the Regional Health Board). Look under FPC or Health in the phone book or ask your local post office or library for a list. Some NHS dentists deal with private patients, too – while others only practise private care and can be found in your local yellow

pages. If you're thinking of changing your dentist, ask neighbours
and friends for recommendations, then telephone and ask for details:
do they provide full NHS preventative care (such as a hygienist),
hours to suit you and an emergency service out of hours? Visit the
surgery and notice if it is clean and tidy, ask about costs for

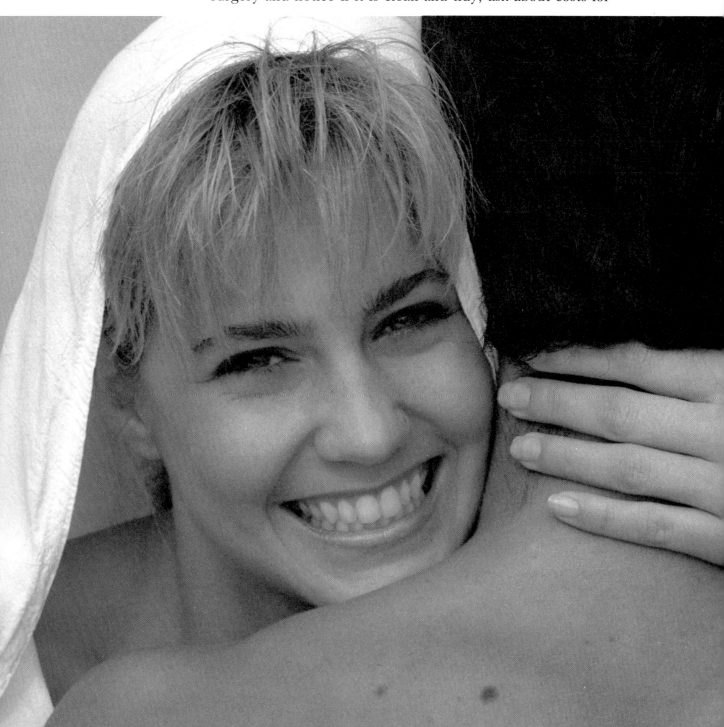

treatment or any special dental services that you or your family may be interested in (teeth crowned, nervous patients, children and so on). Finally, remember that if you're not happy with your dentist, you can easily change to another one. Although dentists don't send on your records, as doctors do, you should ask for your X rays to be transferred or collect them yourself from the surgery.

How do you know if treatment is good? The answer is that you don't, unless your teeth give you trouble. But you may change dentists at any time, without giving a reason.

At the time of writing *NHS check ups* are free but patients are required to contribute towards the cost of each item or treatment performed. Ask your dentist for details. Free treatment is given to young people under 18, or 19 in full-time education (although those over 16 must contribute towards bridges or dentures), expectant mothers or those with a baby under 1 year and those on supplementary benefits or a state pension.

If you have a complaint about NHS treatment from your dentist, first return to the surgery. If this doesn't resolve it, contact your local Family Practitioner Committee or Scottish Health Board (the address is available at your town hall or Regional Council offices) and inform them of the problem within six months of the bad treatment.

Private treatment. Always ask for costs before going ahead with treatments. There are no official bodies to sort out grievances, so if you've received unsatisfactory treatment and your dentist won't help, your only recourse is to consult a solicitor.

If you're afraid of dental treatment tell your dentist. It's a common problem and the dentist may be able to help. Hypnotherapy is sometimes used to calm anxiety. Laughing gas (nitrous oxide and oxygen) allows the patients to stay conscious, but not feel pain. Injections around the relevant tooth numb the area – ask your dentist for them. Dentists will also prescribe tranquillisers to calm down 'phobic' patients before they reach the surgery – but beware, these drugs can be habit forming.

Eyesight

Eyes are the 'windows of the soul'. They reflect character, emotion and health. One of the first things people notice about you, your eyes are one of your best beauty assets. Whether you were born with good or bad eyesight, your eyes serve you every minute of the waking day. They are one of the main keys to the brain and the majority of all information is absorbed through the eye of a sighted person. In some jobs and situations (for example, driving) it is actually an offence to have uncorrected, defective vision. So, by looking after your eyes, you'll be protecting the wonderful enriching sense of sight, boosting a beauty bonus and giving yourself the best opportunity to live life to the full in the future.

Get into the habit of having your own and your family's eyes tested every year (at the time of writing it is free under the NHS and you are not required to buy your spectacles, should you need them, from the same source).

What to watch for: Blurred distance vision (in one or both eyes), inflammation, styes, frequent headaches, dizziness, inability to concentrate on print.

What you'll be tested for: Whether your eyes are functioning and acting as they should. A qualified, registered ophthalmic optician will also be able to detect signs of eye disease and certain health disorders in other parts of your body through your eyes.

What the optician may find: Eyes deteriorate as we get older. Most adults over 45 won't have perfect vision and may need glasses to help them see more clearly. (Nearly half the population in Britain wear some sort of vision correction – either glasses or contact lenses.) If near objects are blurred and distorted and you have difficulty concentrating, you may be told that you are long sighted. Short sightedness is indicated by not being able to see distant objects clearly. Like most parts of the body that go in pairs, one eye may be performing better than the other and a prescription for glasses or contact lenses will take this into account.

Spectacles. Once you have a prescription for your vision requirements, there are several options. If you've decided on glasses, depending on your vision, you'll need to choose the kind of lenses that you'd like. Single vision lenses are the natural choice for anyone who does not require different prescriptions for distance and near vision. Bifocals include two different prescriptions in the same lens. A section (in a wide variety of shapes) allows you clearer near vision, leaving the majority of the lens for distance vision. Trifocals, as the name suggests, also allow another option of vision at arm's length. And varifocals combine gradually increasing power between the different sections of lens.

Next the decision is whether to go for glass or plastic resin based lenses. Glass lenses are usually thinner and scratch less easily than plastic (even though plastic lenses can be coated with a scratch resistant cover). Glass lenses are, on the whole, heavier but can be reinforced to make them less likely to smash in accidents. Children and sports enthusiasts would obviously be better off with plastic lenses for safety's sake.

You can choose whether to have clear or tinted lenses. Tints come in many shades, and graduated tints, where the tint fades gradually from the top of the lens down, are a popular option. Photochromic lenses, which turn darker in sunlight, are available in plastic or glass. An anti-reflection coating stops the 'glassy' look in lenses and allows your eyes to be seen more clearly. Other options are special coloured coatings for VDU operators to minimise glare and anti-fog coatings for sportspeople, preventing misty lenses through contact with water or sweat.

Frames are made in all sorts of materials, colours and shapes. Finding one to suit you can enhance your overall appearance. Children under 16, or 19 in full-time education, along with those claiming certain state benefits, are entitled to vouchers towards new spectacles (the amount depends on what kind of spectacles are needed). Special toughened frames are available for those who play sports such as squash, and there are even underwater diving masks especially made so that they can be fitted with prescription lenses. Ask your optician for details.

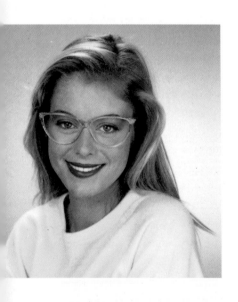

Suit your face by matching your frames to your face shape and hairstyle. A strong, heavy hairstyle will need bold frames to compete and show up your eyes, whereas lighter frames are best for thin or swept back hair. A high bridge on your glasses can make a small nose look longer; whereas a low, heavier bridge disguises a bigger or long nose. Notice if your eyes are close together or far apart – a careful choice of frames can improve your appearance. The top of your frames should be level with your eyebrows, except for half-lens spectacles, of course.

Oval faces suit most shapes. Round faces need balancing at the top part of the face, so opt for angular or square frames which give emphasis and wideness to the top part of the head and make sure the frames are large enough to appear in proportion to the rest of your face. Square jawlines are softened by more rounded or pear shaped frames. Pointed chins with broad foreheads need finer frames to detract from the top face area; choose lighter more neutral colours, too. Long faces look more attractive with heavier and wider, rounded frames, to bring the emphasis sideways instead of down.

Contact lenses. Most people with healthy eyes and normal tear ducts can be fitted with contact lenses and they are generally more efficient than glasses. They float in the fluid in front of the eye giving all-round vision. If you enjoy wearing eye make-up, they need not be a mixed blessing. While you will be able to see more easily to put on make-up (just put your lenses in first), you'll also have to be careful not to get fine powder or mascara filaments in your eye. Foreign bodies in the eye can get trapped under the lens and scratch your delicate eyeball, resulting in inflammation of the eye and making wearing contact lenses uncomfortable. But there are special make-up brands for lens wearers. Generally, if you do decide to opt for lenses, you will need to be scrupulous about the frequency of check-ups and lens care procedures.

Contact lenses come in either hard or soft types. Hard lenses last longer and give slightly better vision. Soft lenses tend to be more comfortable at first. High water content soft lenses can be kept in for longer periods. The new gas permeable hard lenses can be kept in overnight, but they require more care than normal hard ones (regular sterilisation and being left in fluid when out of the eye because they can dry out) and they are more expensive to fit. Nowadays you can be fitted with contact lenses with blue, hazel or green tints – so if you'd like a change of eye colour they'll give you a new shade!

Glare. If you spend a day in bright sunshine you can lose up to 50% of that night's vision. Snow and outside sports enthusiasts, VDU operators, those with early cataracts, albinos, pilots and drivers are just some of the people who ought to be protecting their eyes from too much light. And if you're outside on a sunny day, it's worth protecting your eyes (never look at the sun directly). Although the eye can recover from most forms of glare, too much or too strong light can damage it permanently. So invest in a good pair of tinted prescription glasses (if you normally wear spectacles) or sunglasses (if you have good eyesight or wear contact lenses). Choose a lens that suits your requirements. All sunglasses protect from glare by cutting down light as it passes through their lenses. Some protect more than others, and your optician will advise on the transmission characteristics of different types.

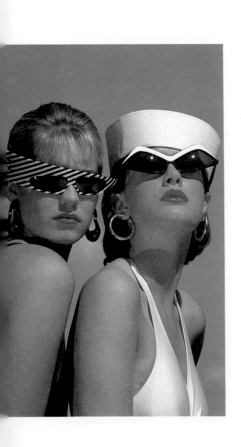

Acrylic plastic lenses can cut out up to 95 per cent of ultraviolet light, depending on the amount of pigment in them. They include plastics such as CR39 or UV96 and are usually the least expensive to buy. These lenses are more prone to scratching than glass but not so likely to break. The tint can be graduated.

Polarised lenses consist of several layers of plastic and/or glass. The polarised formation blocks out the horizontal waves of UV light (seen as white glare), and instead allows a more vertical light wave through so that wearers can see shade and colour. Lenses can be mirrored or graded from light to dark.

Photochromic lenses work on a photo-negative basis with built-in light sensitive crystals that become darker as the light outside gets brighter and vice versa. As they always look light indoors, it's wise to take them into daylight before buying to see how quickly, and how dark, they become.

Mirrored glasses can be polarised or acrylic coated with a special reflector. Some only allow 15 per cent of light through, so choose carefully for driving or sport where you may need to see more detail.

Defective lenses can distort a wearer's vision and so can be dangerous for driving. They may even cause headaches. To check for defects, hold the sunglasses at arm's length and look at a vertical object through each lens in turn, then gently rotate them. If the line 'kinks' the lens is faulty.

Grey or brown tints are suitable for most purposes. Brightly coloured lenses will distort colour perception, so don't wear them for driving.

Don't choose a dark tint for Britain. As the light rarely becomes very bright you need only a pale to medium tint for good visibility and to cut down glare.

Stick to well-known manufacturers. Cheaper 'fashion' sunglasses can do more damage than good. Don't wear sunspecs indoors and take them off in shade. Aim to wear them only when glare makes your eyes water badly.

Sports people may wish to opt for added side lenses, to cut out glare. But this will also reduce side vision. Ear clips are ideal for activity, goggle lenses for watersport enthusiasts.

Sunbathers should seek out eye-shaped shades which are best for maximum tan and protection, but make sure the lens covers the eye up to the eyebrow and so protects this delicate area. Use a sunscreen on the skin of the eye area as UV light can bounce in at other angles.

Drivers need plastic lenses that don't shatter and so are safer than glass in accidents. Polarised lenses can cause distortion if you've also got a polarised windscreen. Graduated lenses make looking down at the dashboard easier. Never wear sunglasses when visibility is poor or it's getting dark. Take them off in tunnels. Don't wear lenses that are too dark.

OTHER EYE PROBLEMS

Conjunctivitis is an eye inflammation in which the membranes around the eye become red, sore and sometimes itchy. It can be caused by deposits in the eye (an eyelash, grit, etc). Try blowing your nose hard and blinking. If this doesn't work, see your doctor or go to the casualty ward of a local hospital immediately. Alternatively conjunctivitis may be caused by hayfever, contact with a germ (steer clear of other people's towels or contact lens solutions, for this reason). Alcohol, late nights and smoky atmospheres may also be reflected by the whites of your eye. In Britain try bathing them with cool tap water; in other countries tap water isn't so safe; instead try an eye wash, available from the chemist. If these don't work, visit your doctor for treatment.

Eyestrain can be caused by concentrating on small print for too long. This won't damage your vision, but it is worth having your eyesight checked to find out if you need visual aid for reading.

Glaucoma or tunnel vision is symptomised by headaches, blurred vision, loss of sideways vision and a feeling of tension in the eye. It is caused by the fluid between the cornea and lens not draining properly, with the canal which drains the area becoming blocked. Milder cases are difficult to diagnose as the eye starts to overcompensate and vision worsens gradually. For less severe cases, treatment is usually by drugs, in eyedrop form. Bad glaucoma may be gradual or sudden, and extreme cases can result in blindness. Surgery to cure glaucoma sometimes includes laser treatment.

Blepharitis is an irritation to the edge of the eyelid, where it becomes sore, dry and flaky. The cause is either allergy or a type of dandruff. Your doctor can prescribe an anti-bacterial eye ointment, if it's appropriate.

Cataract. In this condition the eye's lens becomes opaque; an operation is necessary for correction.

Detached retina is where the lens inside the eye (the retina) comes away from the eyeball and requires sealing by an operation. (Many of these operations are now being done by laser for pin-point accuracy.)

Styes are inflammation of the eyelid and similar to a boil. Bathe them in warm water and treat with special preparations available from a chemist.

Blocked tear ducts need a doctor's help. Visit one straight away.

EYE CARE

Look after your eyes by treating them with tender loving care. Never rub them, be careful with eye make-up removal (use a tissue, rather than cotton wool, which consists of small filaments that can get trapped in the eye), rest them as often as possible, always protect them from glare (on sunbeds *always* make sure you wear protective goggles), make sure you read or work in a good light (daylight is ideal but if your office has neon strip lighting, ask your employers for a more restful light to avoid eye strain and headaches). VDU operators should ask for expert advice on positioning of their computers for least eye strain. (Green script is believed to be more restful on the eyes than white.)

EYE EXERCISE

Although eye exercises cannot cure imperfect vision, just as with any other part of the body they help supply blood and firm up muscles around the eye. This helps to keep the eye healthier and in good working order. Try blinking as much as possible, especially when concentrating (for example, on a computer screen or television) and in dry atmospheres (planes, for instance) where the eye can dry and become sore and irritated. Get your eyes into focus first thing in the morning by blinking slowly 20 times (a useful time to do this is when you're brushing your teeth). Also spend some time rolling your eyes round in a clockwise, then anticlockwise direction. Then try darting your glance from side to side and from a distant object to a close one. Aim to spend a few minutes doing your eye exercises every day and you'll find it helps eyes to look clearer and makes them feel brighter.

Aches and pains

Aches and pains are nature's way of telling you that something is wrong. So be your own bodyguard and stake them out with a round the body guide. After all, a diagnosis is the first step to recovery.

Please remember: If a pain is sharp or sudden, goes on for longer than 24 hours without getting better or you can't find the cause, go and see your doctor.

What is pain? A local or more general sensation ranging from discomfort to agony, caused by stimulation of nerve endings; it is a protective mechanism. An *ache* is dull, throbbing, constant pain.

HEAD

Headaches can result from allergies, stress, tiredness, bad diet, eye strain, too much sun or alcohol or, as you get older, when arteries thicken or blood pressure is high. Enlarged blood vessels, pressing on nerves or contracting muscles in the head, are the cause. Headaches can be relieved with one of the many painkillers on the market but if you suffer from regular headaches, go to your doctor for advice.

Migraine is said to affect up to six million people in Britain and it's more common in women. Theories on causes cover hormonal changes, certain foods, visual or physical changes (such as a flickering TV or change of climate), stress and hereditary factors. Migraines can last for hours or sometimes days, and like allergies they may suddenly start or, better, stop. *Common migraine* often includes nausea and vomiting, too. *Classic migraine* sufferers experience other symptoms, such as visual disturbances, intolerance to light and noise and tingling in limbs. A doctor may prescribe a long-term preventative drug or one to take when an attack is threatened. Some migraine drugs, such as ergotamine tartrate, come in suppository, inhaled or soluble forms. Your GP may refer you to a neurological clinic for further help. For those who like natural remedies, feverfew is believed to help relieve suffering.

Sinusitis or antritis is infection and pain of the sinuses or antrum cavities in the mid forehead and cheeks. Occurring usually after a cold, they can be treated with antibiotics. Regular sufferers may require a 'washout' operation to clear the cavity and prevent recurrence.

Earache should be dealt with quickly, as the thin auditory membrane, the eardrum, is easily damaged by infection and deafness can result. See your doctor.

Toothache sufferers will want to get help fast! Applied oil of cloves or painkillers may help dampen down the offending nerve until you reach your dentist.

Head injuries should always be checked by a doctor for fractures or concussion, especially if there is loss of consciousness, faintness and pain.

NECK

If you look at the skeleton, you'll see that the neck is a very thin layer of bones, joining a rather heavy skull to the body. No wonder necks sometimes complain! Tension shows in the neck as a small ball, where the neck meets the skull. Sleeping at an awkward angle, bad posture and draughts also cause aches and pains here. Heat and gentle massage can help relieve them. Arthritis can start in the spine at the back of the neck (see Back/Spine/Hips section).

SHOULDER

Frozen shoulders (inflammation of tissue) should be rested, massaged and given heat treatments. But if you injure your shoulder where it meets the arm and it shows no sign of getting better, it may be damaged – go and see your doctor.

ABDOMEN/ STOMACH

Heart attacks and *indigestion* are sometimes mistaken for each other. A *heart attack* is pain in the middle of the chest, with symptoms such as clamminess, faintness and tingling down the left arm and it's made worse by exercise. *Indigestion* or *heartburn* is again mid-chest pain but other symptoms such as an acid taste in the mouth, flatulence and wind show that it is a gastric problem. Indigestion is made worse by bending or lying down but can be relieved by drinking water with some bicarbonate of soda.

Ulcers cause a burning pain before eating (often called 'hunger pains') or after. You should see your doctor for treatment.

Pain at the side of the abdomen may be a *hernia*, where the intestine bulges through a weakness in the muscle and shows as a swelling, or it may be a *pulled muscle* (seek your doctor's advice).

Another common confusion is between *womb* and *bowel* pain. Womb pain may be related to *menstruation*; other symptoms such as irregular bleeding or discharge should be checked out by your doctor.

Constipation, when painful, requires a mild laxative or a rethink of your diet to include more bran or roughage foods. If constipation occurs regularly (apart from before a period, when it is common), visit your doctor.

One of the most common causes of abdominal pain is *irritable bowel syndrome* which is believed to affect over 20 per cent of the population at some time in their lives. Pain can be chronic. Under this syndrome come symptoms such as spastic colon, mucus colitis, constipation, diarrhoea, nausea, wind, adhesions, distension of the stomach and pain. Doctors don't know the cause but believe that it's diet linked. Those under stress or recovering from an illness or operation are more likely to suffer.

Other pains to watch out for in the abdomen are caused by *gall* and *kidney stones*, *pancreatitis* and chronic inflammations. Be on guard for the acute pain that indicates haemorrhaging in an ovarian cyst, ectopic (tubal) pregnancy or an appendicitis (these are in the lower abdomen, pelvic region).

Herpes is a viral infection characterised by pain and tingling before the blister or rash occurs. Herpes zoster is *shingles* and a rash occurs over the body. Herpes can also occur as *cold sores* on the mouth or around the *genital* area and are easily transmitted to others by touch. Take painkillers and see your doctor for advice on treatment.

BACK/SPINE/HIPS

Back pain is the major cause of days off work in Britain. Apart from the arthritis complaints detailed below, pain from the top of your neck to the base of your spine may be caused by bad posture (see Chapter 6), overweight (especially big breasts), unsupportive chairs, restrictive clothing, constant bending (e.g. gardening) or a bad mattress (see the sleep section, Chapter 10). Stress and strains may be to your spinal column or muscles and in surrounding tissue. Treat with rest, heat and massage. Painkillers and deep heat sprays also help to relieve aches and pain.

Rheumatism means inflammation and pain in bones, muscles or surrounding tissues or joints. Twenty million people suffer from rheumatism each year and there are many different types of rheumatoid diseases. Some people have a once only attack.

Arthritis is a disease of the joints and the most common forms are *rheumatoid* and *osteo*.

Rheumatoid arthritis is inflammation of connective tissue and affects three times as many women as men, usually starting in the thirties. It is rarely found in the hips or spine but can cause inflammation in joint linings and around the heart or lung. Rheumatoid arthritis tends to suddenly flare up and die away.

Osteoarthritis is the more widespread damage to the surface of the joint bones. It develops with age and often starts after the menopause, also affecting more women than men. Osteoarthritis is made much worse by being overweight. Any joint in the body may

suffer from osteoarthritis, usually diagnosed by stiffening, swelling
and painful joints – but knees, hands, feet and fingers, as well as top
of the spine and hips are particularly prone. It's worth trying aspirin
and getting advice from your GP immediately, if you suspect you
have arthritis. S/he may give you drugs to prevent deterioration,
surgery in bad cases (for example, hip or knee replacements) or
refer you to a physiotherapist for exercises to help mobility.
Collagen injections (see Cosmetic Surgery section in this chapter)
have been used to relieve some painful joints – but always check
with your GP first. Some sufferers swear by homoeopathic
medicines or copper bracelets as remedies but there is no medical
evidence to support their use.

Osteoporosis is the gradual loss of calcium in the bones from
which both men and women suffer as they get older. Although HRT
(hormone replacement therapy) will allay the loss and thinning of
bones in women, when treatment stops or after the menopause
average loss is around one per cent of bone matter a year. The most
common results are fractures in the wrist or hip and spinal crush
fractures (shown as the distinctive 'dowager's hump'). One in two
women suffer some sort of bone fracture problem by the age of 70.
Unfortunately the need for hip replacement operations is common
and may require a long wait on the NHS. Although osteoporosis
can't be prevented altogether, and taking extra calcium later in life
doesn't make up for the loss, you should make sure you stock up on
calcium and maintain healthy bones with regular exercise at a
younger age. Smoking and not eating enough dairy produce lead to
less calcium being absorbed by the body. And if you're small boned
and of slim build, it might be worth revising your diet to make sure
you receive increased calcium and/or take a calcium supplement,
too.

Lumbago is a general term for backache in the lumber (lower
spine) area. *Sciatica* is usually tingling and pain in the lower back,
thighs or legs. Sciatica is used as a general term to cover pressure of
a disc (vertebra) on a nerve, as well as inflammation of the sciatic
nerve in the lower back. A *slipped* or *herniated* disc is when the
nucleus of a vertebral pad protrudes out into the surrounding tissue
and presses on spinal nerves.

More conventional medicine is beginning to recognise nowadays
that so-called 'alternative' therapists can help some joint and spine
problems. Osteopathy is manipulation of the joints and spine to treat

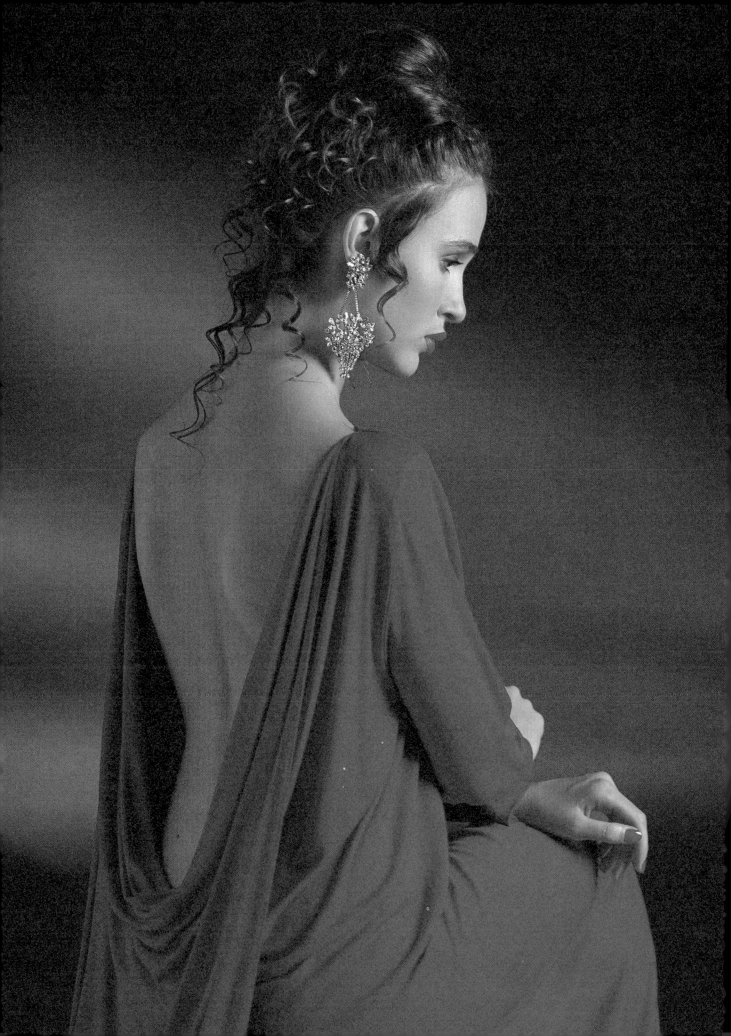

disorders here and related nervous conditions. Chiropractors concentrate mainly on the spine and often use X rays for diagnosis.

LIMBS

Varicose veins have weakened walls and so dilate to cause problems. They can be relieved by rest, wearing support tights but not high heels. Injections or surgery from a doctor may seal or remove them.

Haemorrhoids or *piles* are varicose veins of the anus. Chemists stock ointments to relieve discomfort and reduce inflammation. Surgery is now more streamlined and advisable for bad sufferers.

Cramp can be caused by lack of calcium or salt, or by constriction of circulation when muscles are out of condition or cold. Pull your toes towards you for relief of cramp in the calves.

Pins and needles are caused by pressure on nerves and usually relieved by movement.

Housemaid's or water on the knee is swelling of the protective pad over the knee cap and pain due to pressure. If it doesn't dispel with rest, visit your doctor.

Tennis elbow is a small muscle tear or bursitis (fluid swelling) of the joint which can occur in the same way as housemaid's knee or be due to excessive and energetic use of the joint.

Sprains usually become stiff, swollen and painful. Make sure a torn or sprained ligament isn't a bone fracture (an X ray will diagnose this) and treat with cold compresses, support bandages and rest. Doctors may give cortisone injections to bad or chronic sprains.

Inflammations, unlike sprains, can occur without injury in ligaments and tendons. Anti-inflammatory drugs along with support and gentle exercises are recommended.

The body heals *bruising* with time.

PAINKILLERS

Aspirin helps to reduce inflammation (for example for rheumatoid arthritis) as well as relieving pain, but don't continually take higher doses or take them on an empty stomach as they can irritate the stomach lining. Paracetamol reduces pain but won't affect inflammation. Codeine is a weaker pain reliever and may cause constipation, if you tend to suffer. Try a 'freeze' aerosol for muscular aches and sprains. Support bandages for elbow, knee, ankle and wrist help reinforce weak or existing injuries and prevent new ones.

———
Exclusively for women

Vaginal problems can cause extreme embarrassment as well as discomfort. But don't be afraid of going to your doctor – he or she will have come across it all before.

If you are shy of seeing a male doctor, ask the receptionist if there is a woman doctor in the practice whom you might see on this occasion. Many surgeries now ask if you'd prefer to see a woman if, for instance, you're going along for a routine smear test. Otherwise ring one of the larger hospitals in your area and ask for an appointment at their 'special' problems or genito-urinary clinic. You don't have to give your own or your doctor's name and address, so the check-up can be completely anonymous, if you wish.

SMEAR TEST

This is when a spatula painlessly takes a few cells, via the vagina, from the outside of the neck of the cervix (womb). These are then studied in a laboratory for signs of abnormal cells. A change in these usually normal cells to becoming cancerous is a slow process, and any abnormality in your smear test may simply be evidence of an infection (even if you're not aware of it). In this case, you'll be given antibiotics and asked to return for another smear test in a few months' time. If the second smear test still shows abnormal cells, you will be referred to a gynaecologist for further tests and possibly treatment.

The advantage of regular smear tests is that they will show up cells which may become cancerous later. Womb (cervical) cancer is completely curable, if it's diagnosed soon enough. Ideally any woman who is sexually active should have a smear test every year, or, at the very least, every two to three years. GPs are prepared to test women over 35 more regularly, as this is the most at-risk group. However cervical cancer is increasing in those of a younger age, so however old you are, ask your doctor regularly for a smear test. Family Planning and genito-urinary clinics will also do them.

DISCHARGE FROM THE VAGINA

Some discharge is normal so long as it isn't blood-stained, smelly or making you itchy or sore. If it is, see a doctor as soon as possible.

Thrush is the most likely cause, a fungal infection usually aggravated by hormonal activity (the Pill, pregnancy), diabetes, taking antibiotics or using perfumed body products. Thrush is not always caught from a sexual partner but it *is* contagious, so it's wise to use a condom or refrain from sexual intercourse until it has cleared. Prevent recurrence by wearing cotton knickers (and avoiding close-fitting jeans or tights), using unperfumed soaps and wiping from front to back after going to the toilet. Your doctor may prescribe antibacterials; some regular sufferers swear by the application of plain yoghurt on to the affected area. Your sexual partner may also need treatment, if thrush recurs, as he may carry the infection and be reinfecting you. Other discharges from the vagina may be due to non-specific urethritis (NSU) or VD. See your doctor for treatment

CYSTITIS

The symptoms of cystitis are the need to pass water, even where there is little urine to pass; a burning, stinging sensation when you do; pain in the lower abdomen; often feverishness and sometimes blood in the urine. It is caused by inflammation of the bladder or urethra through infection, bruising (through sexual intercourse, horse or bicycle riding; the so-called 'honeymoon' cystitis), allergy to washing powder, contraceptives, perfumed bath products or a reaction to spicy foods or strong drinks. As four out of five women suffer from cystitis at some time in their lives, there is no need to worry; but first-time sufferers should (and will probably want to) go straight to the doctor for treatment. S/he may suggest a urine test to establish which type of bacteria is causing the condition and make sure these aren't symptoms of a more serious disease. Your chemist can offer immediate over-the-counter treatment before an appointment. Regular sufferers should take the same precautions as thrush sufferers, while also making sure that they pass water up to 15 minutes after sexual intercourse. During a bout of cystitis, drink plenty of water to 'flush' out infection, dilute concentrated urine and allow you to pass urine more frequently.

PRE-MENSTRUAL TENSION

At some time in their lives one in three women suffer from pre-menstrual tension. These are the symptoms of hormonal change after ovulation each month. PMT occurs from fourteen to a couple of days before a period. Symptoms include sore breasts, skin disorders, bloating, appetite cravings, headaches, depression, irritability, dizziness, tiredness, loss of sex drive and others. The 'syndrome' (as it's now called because tension is not the only symptom) is now recognised, on the whole, by GPs. It can vary from being mildly inconvenient to disrupting the sufferer's normal life. Although why it happens is not completely understood, doctors often prescribe diuretics (for water retention) or sometimes hormones or tranquillisers. First, though, you should try self help with a course of vitamin B_6 (50mg twice a day) and magnesium or evening primrose oil and zinc supplements, starting three days before symptoms usually occur. Your local chemist or health store will carry products containing these trace nutrients made especially for pre-menstrual tension. And try natural herbal diuretics, celery or cucumber, if bloating is the problem. Diet is important too; try cutting down on animal fats and step up fibre. Reduce caffeine intake and take small, regular meals to make sure you keep your blood sugar level up. If this doesn't work, bad sufferers may wish to ask their doctor for further help – perhaps a prescribed course of hormone treatment.

PERIODS

Menstruation should not restrict your normal lifestyle. Some religions still impose restrictions on women who are menstruating but this is becoming rather old fashioned in the Western world. Periods should not stop you exercising, washing your hair, touching milk (it won't turn sour, as believed by old wives), having sexual intercourse (if you and your partner wish to), or swimming (with the aid of tampons). Exercise is good for menstrual cramps, which affect some women more than others. Called dysmenorrhoea, painful periods can be eased with drugs available from the chemist and made especially for the purpose. One type of dysmenorrhea is reduced after childbirth, but unfortunately another type appears to worsen with age and isn't affected by having a baby. If symptoms are severe (not eased by the recommended dose of painkillers from the chemist) or prolonged, visit your doctor for further advice.

Changes in bleeding. Menstrual cycles differ from woman to woman. A cycle of anywhere between 21 to 35 days is usual, but some women are regularly irregular! Bleeding lasting for a week is as normal for one woman as a three-day period for another.

Heaviness of bleeding differs, too – often it will change following stress, travel or hormonal activity. But if you suddenly stop menstruating, start bleeding between periods or find that you're suffering from extra heavy blood loss for no apparent reason, it is worth going to your doctor. Causes can be as simple as a course of drugs, pregnancy or an over-enthusiastic slimming regime. But as the symptoms can indicate more dangerous diseases, it is worthwhile putting your mind at rest. Your doctor may suggest a D & C (dilation and curette) to remove and examine tissue in the womb. Done under general anaesthetic, this operation requires half a day in hospital and is not painful.

MENOPAUSE

The average age for the change of life ranges from 45 to 59, but some women experience it older or even go through it in their 30s. There is no way of predicting when you will experience the menopause or what the symptoms will be. Two out of 10 women say that they have very few problems – their periods become irregular and then eventually cease. Side effects are minimal and they are relieved at no longer having pre-menstrual tension or worrying about contraception. (Wait for one year after your last period if over 50 or two years if under 50 before ceasing contraception.) But sometimes irregular bleeding can continue from three to ten years, along with symptoms such as hot flushes, swelling, night sweating, giddiness, headaches, mood swings. Sex becomes difficult as the vagina is drier and there is more risk of genito-urinary infections.

This all happens because the ovaries and other organs have stopped producing the hormones necessary for pregnancy. And changes occur – it is mainly a lack of oestrogen which causes the less pleasant symptoms. Take a positive approach by getting enough rest and exercise, maintaining a healthy (and non-fattening) diet, reducing your salt intake if you suffer from water retention and making sure you wear a good supportive bra. Be scrupulous about personal hygiene. If you are suffering from hot flushes and sweating you may feel more comfortable taking two showers a day. Also do explain your symptoms to your family so that they will understand what is happening to you and offer reassurance and support if you experience depression.

If the symptoms of menopause are making your and/or your family's life a misery, or if you are suffering from heavy bleeding, go and see your doctor. S/he may prescribe tranquillisers for problems with sleeping and irritability (take them only if these are severe and view them as a temporary measure), diuretics for water retention and oestrogen creams for vaginal dryness. A doctor may also suggest referring you to a gynaecologist or put you on HRT (hormone replacement therapy). With careful calculations of the right dose of oestrogen and progestogen for the individual, many women who suffer severe problems have benefited from HRT. Some women at risk from serious illnesses are not suitable for HRT and will have to rely on their own health knowledge and the doctor's advice.

HRT usually consists of tablets similar to the Pill (although they do *not* act as a contraceptive) and you will experience monthly bleeding just as before the menopause started. Some gynaecologists will do an implant: a 'pellet' is implanted in the groin area to slowly release the hormonal drugs needed over six months. This takes a few seconds under local anaesthetic and is painless. Length of treatments varies from six months to several years. There is also a new stick-on patch to release the HRT through the skin's surface.

Finally, remember that the menopause is natural and does pass. If you are suffering from bad or unpleasant symptoms, they won't go on for ever (the average 'change' is around two years). And although everyone should take greater care of their health as they get older, there is no reason why you should not be as happy and fulfilled and feel as fit as ever.

BREASTS

Taking care of your breasts is an investment in your looks, your health and possibly your baby's health (if you breast feed). Basically breasts, or mammary glands as they're clinically called, are there to produce milk to feed offspring. All mammals have them, though humans in the Western world are peculiar in finding them important sexually. (In parts of Africa, for instance, breasts are used to point at something or putting a hand on someone's breast may be a form of greeting.) But returning to the scientific: breasts develop at puberty and consist of fatty tissue, protecting milk glands which run in a duct system to the nipple. Breasts contain no muscle and are supported against gravity by ligaments under them, on the chest wall. Nipples consist of erectile tissue and so harden to tactile influences such as touch and cold, or emotional ones such as sexual excitement. Hormonal changes in the body affect breasts. The main ones are the Pill, pregnancy or just before a period when breasts can become swollen and tender. Some drugs will affect them, too; your doctor should warn you.

So why do men have them? No one knows. But men's breasts are of the same structure as females' and they *can* suffer from the same breast problems.

The Pill. While doctors argue about the association of breast growths with progestogens in the Pill, the Family Planning Association has advised clinics to stop prescribing some types which are absorbed at a higher rate. As high oestrogen pills are reported to have other side effects, it's wise to opt for a combined low dosage one. Some find that the Pill makes breasts sore and swollen for the first month or so of taking; if this continues after three months, ask for a change of prescription. After the birth of a baby, some combined pills can dry up or decrease nutrients in breast milk and are best avoided if you are breast feeding.

Support. Whether or not to wear a bra should be determined by comfort and size of breasts. Anyone over a 34B cup would be advised to do so from day to day. Special sports bras are a must (minimum stretch and well separated cups control bounce best) to avoid 'jogger's nipples', and these can also be helpful for pre-menstruation or Pill-swollen breasts too. A well-fitting maternity bra minimises stretch marks and sagging from extra weight and you may find it more comfortable to sleep in one, too, though breasts may never be quite the same after pregnancy and breast feeding. Two or three new bras each year are necessary to give enough regular support as elastic loses its stretch with washing. Underwired bras give the best support for big breasts and also make more of smaller ones. Wire is finer and more comfortable than it used to be. Manufacturers say that the average breast size is going up from 34B to 36B.

To find your fit. Over your present bra but without top clothes, measure just under breasts, where the fabric meets the flesh. Add five inches for your *bra size* (taking the larger measurement if the size is in between). For *cup size* measure around the fullest part of your bust. The same as your bra size means that you're an A cup; go up a cup for every extra inch (for example, 2″ more than 34″ – i.e. 36″ – is bra size 34C). When trying on a bra, put on the straps first and lean forwards to allow your breasts to fill the cups. Then fasten the back. Adjust the straps so that nipples are parallel with mid upper arm. You should be able to slip a finger under the midriff line and two fingers under each strap. A well fitting bra shouldn't mark when you take it off after a few minutes. Take a T-shirt with you to put over the top and check for bulge lines.

Shape and size. It's normal, as with hands, feet and eyes, for one breast to be slightly larger than the other. But as they don't contain muscle, it's difficult to change breast shape. Breasts consist mainly of fat; losing *some* weight will reduce the size but it won't affect the firmness (quick large weight loss can leave sagging breasts). Good posture keeps the supporting muscles working; correct yours by relaxing shoulders down and back as you inhale, pulling in your stomach and imagining a string pulling you up from the top of your head.

Bust toning lotions and creams, along with *massage* or *cold baths* may improve surface texture but won't make any difference to the uplift or overall shape. *Exercise* will. It firms up the support muscles. One of the best is swimming (crawl and back stroke, too) or pretending to swim on dry land. Feel the muscles working by standing straight with feet slightly apart; press palms of hands together in front of you as though praying (elbows out) and press hard as you inhale, relax in as you exhale. Repeat while stepping up speed. Or clasp your hands behind your back and, without moving arms or shoulders, press hands down into the small of your back as you inhale; relax as you exhale and repeat.

Apart from hormonal influences the only other way to change your shape is by surgery (see Cosmetic Surgery section).

Nipples vary from woman to woman in shape, size and site. *Slight discharge* may be due to hormonal changes, and is sometimes normal during the latter half of the menstrual cycle; but seek your doctor's advice if worried and especially if the discharge is bloodstained or occurs after the menopause. *Inverted nipples*, although more prone to infection, aren't abnormal, unless one suddenly inverts. Breast shields from the chemist and massage can help revert them for breast feeding. *A rash* present only on the nipple should be taken seriously if it is chronic (see your doctor). *Hair* here is best dealt with by a qualified electrolysist, depilatory cream (check for allergy) or individual plucking in the direction that the hair is growing and after a bath when pores are wider. *Skin* on nipples is sensitive; protect it with a high protection sunscreen if sunbathing topless.

Breast problems. Nine out of ten lumps found in breasts are not harmful. But breast cancer is one of the highest causes of deaths in women and completely curable if caught early enough. So it's well worthwhile for every woman over 16 to check her breasts each month. The best time is the week following a period. Most at risk from breast cancer are those with more than one close relative who's had it; least likely candidates are the under 25s who've had a baby.

Do the breast test. Lie on your back on a flat surface with your head on a pillow and left shoulder slightly raised by a folded towel. Feel the left breast with the flat fingers, held together, of the right hand. Press the breast gently but firmly in towards the body. Work in a spiral, from the nipple. Feel every part. With your left arm above your head, and elbow bent, repeat the spiral carefully. Make sure you carefully feel the outer part of the breast. Finish by feeling the tail of the breast towards the armpit. Repeat all stages on the other breast. Be thorough and don't rush. Do the test every month.

Most lumps are fibrous tissue (harmless thickening of the tissue) or cysts (where liquid secreted by milk glands does not drain away through ducts). Often lumps appear just before a period and disappear afterwards. Larger, individual cysts are free moving under the skin and can be drained or surgically removed, if troublesome.

Mastitis is an inflammation of the milk ducts, showing as painful lumpiness, often pre-menstrually. A supportive bra helps comfort. Infectious mastitis can occur when breast feeding and responds to draining and/or antibiotics.

Rashes may be caused by heat under heavy breasts, so make sure you dry thoroughly after washing. Or rashes may be caused by an allergy to soap powders.

LUMP TREATMENTS

If there's any doubt, your doctor will arrange for a mammography or xerography X ray (thermography, the heat X ray, is less specific and not so popular these days). S/he may decide to do a biopsy to test for malignancy by draining some fluid from the lump, usually under local anaesthetic, or removing the lump under general anaesthetic (a lumpectomy). These days surgeons believe in telling a patient when the lump is cancerous before operating further. A woman should not be asked to agree to a mastectomy before she goes in for a lumpectomy. Experts say that a delay of up to a month makes little difference to the tumour and can allow the patient to come to terms with the diagnosis, while considering the options for treatments.

Partial mastectomy is where the lump and surrounding tissue are removed leaving some of the breast. *Simple mastectomy* is where the breast is removed. *Radical mastectomy* is now rarely considered necessary but involves removing the breast and the surrounding area, including lymph glands under the arm.

Treatments that may help protect you further. Local radiation is applied with radioactive wires inserted into the area around the cancer during the operation and left for two to three days. Chemotherapy or anti-oestrogen treatment after the operation helps stop the cancer spread, especially in post-menopausal women. Anti-oestrogen treatment may also be given to those whose cancer is too advanced for local treatment.

Evidence has shown that those diagnosed by screening units have an earlier and better chance of cure and safe treatment for breast cancer. Experts would like the government to spend more money on establishing nationwide screening because of the potential for saving lives. In the long term this could also result in an economic benefit, since less women would require expensive treatment for advanced breast cancer. The Breast Care and Mastectomy Association supplies aftercare advice to hospitals or individuals from volunteers, who have all had mastectomies. Contact them at 26 Harrison Street, London WC1H 8JG, tel: 01 837 0908, for further information.

Pregnancy

Before becoming pregnant get into tip-top shape to give your baby the best start in life. Pay special attention to healthy eating and your weight. Being overweight could reduce your chances of conception. And don't forget your partner – the healthier he is, the better equipped to deal with your pregnancy. Those with complaints such as heart disease, epilepsy or diabetes should seek advice from their doctor before trying to conceive. If there is a family history of hereditary illness (for example 'Down's syndrome', sickle cell disease, thalassaemia, muscular dystrophy, Huntingdon's chorea or haemophilia) ask your doctor to refer you to a genetic counsellor.

At least three months before conceiving, make *sure* that you're immune to German measles (rubella); your doctor will test and immunise, if necessary.

When you first know stop taking any drugs (e.g. travel sickness or analgesics). Check with your doctor or pharmacist immediately if you are prescribed medication.

Don't alter your diet so long as it's balanced, with plenty of milk and dairy products, fresh fruit, vegetables and proteins (pulses, lean meats, fish). If your diet isn't all it should be, you may consider supplementing with multi-vitamin and minerals (iron and folic acid, especially). And if you don't eat dairy products ask your doctor about taking calcium supplements.

Cut to a minimum, or stop, smoking and drinking alcohol. Avoid excess caffeine. Try not to stand for long periods and sit down immediately if you feel faint.

Take pleasure in your pregnancy but carry on as normal, if all is well. Basically, anything that is not good for you out of pregnancy, isn't good for you in it.

The first three months. Pregnancies vary in character. Morning sickness affects most (but not all) women (and some sympathetic husbands!) and it may not just be in the morning. Dry biscuits and cups of tea may help. Doctors can prescribe a drug to ease extreme cases. You may find you 'go off' certain foods and crave others. Avoid constipation by taking plenty of fluids and dried or raw fruit (a natural laxative). Feeling tired is common – make time for more rest. Be sure to see your doctor at eight to 12 weeks, so that you are referred to ante-natal classes.

The middle three months. At 12 to 16 weeks go to ante-natal classes. Here you'll find support, advice and the answer to any worries. You'll be asked to return every fourth week until your 28th week of pregnancy; after this at two-weekly intervals until the 36th week and then weekly until the baby is born. These times are under review as many feel they are too frequent. Sickness, breast tingling and tiredness will *usually* have settled by the twelfth week. And your doctor will now feel safer prescribing you necessary drugs. By the fifth month you'll find waistbands don't fit and the baby starts to kick. Women over 35 may opt for an amniocentesis test in the 16th to 18th week and the period of rest afterwards varies from individual to individual.

The last three months. From the 17th week your baby is almost fully formed. Blood pressure and samples are taken regularly. Weight and swelling will be carefully monitored.

Diet and weight gain. Most doctors believe you should gain 20 to

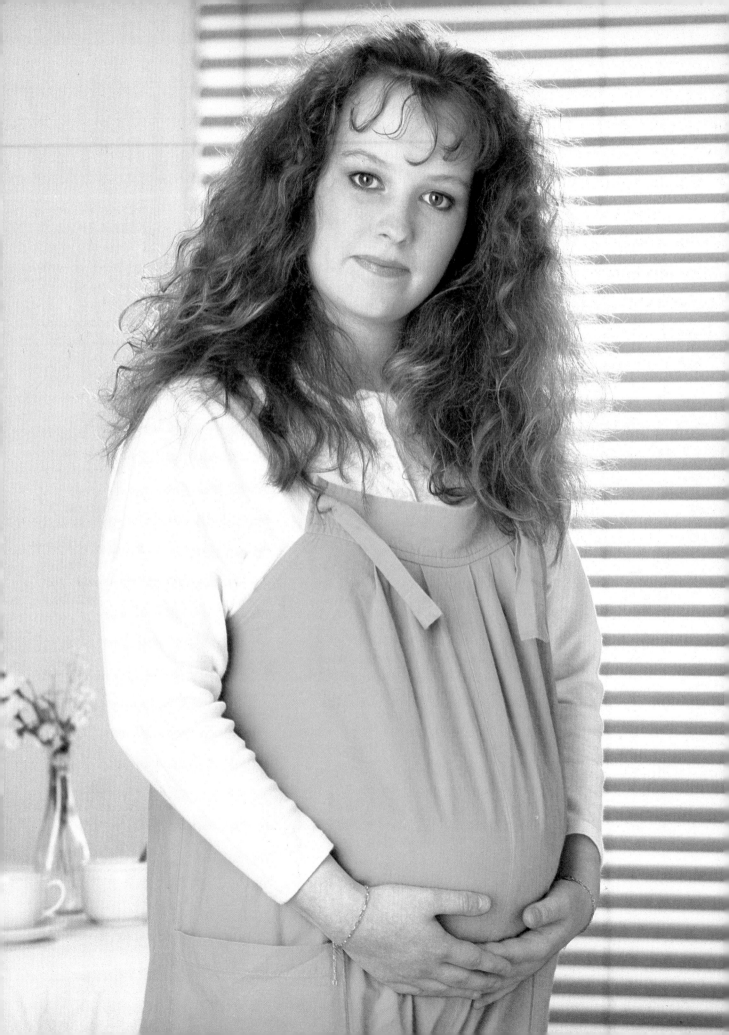

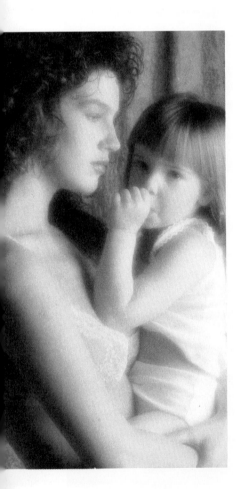

30lbs (9 to 13½k) during a 40-week pregnancy, but not everyone does. It is important not to be overweight. The extra weight (mainly around stomach, tops of thighs, bottom and breasts) consists of the baby, amniotic fluid, placenta and fat store for breast feeding. If you don't breast feed, you should aim to be back to normal weight between six weeks and three months after delivery. Nursing mothers may find that they can't get back to shape until they cease breast feeding. As far as diet goes during pregnancy, *don't* eat for two. Your energy intake should be around 3,000 calories a day, that's 500 more than normal. By the end of the third month your daily diet should include bodybuilding foods such as half to one pint of milk, fish or lean meat, salads or green vegetables, cheese or butter.

Exercise. Continue sports such as swimming, cycling, tennis if they're part of a standard exercise programme and your pregnancy is normal. But cut down on strenuous activities such as jogging and squash. Ask your doctor, if you're not sure. Ante-natal classes will suggest exercises to help keep you supple and prepare you for childbirth.

Stretch marks. No one knows why they sometimes occur. We *do* know that creams, lotions, oils and promises won't prevent them and that they fade gradually. A moisturising cream will help skin-stretch damage and make taut tummies feel more comfortable and less itchy.

Skin. Some women look their best during pregnancy with a dazzling complexion and glowing shiny hair. Others find hormonal activity wreaks havoc on their looks. Many pregnant women suffer from deeper pigmentation (chloasma) such as 'the mask of pregnancy' over cheeks or deepening colour of scars, but these can be disguised by a covering foundation. New spider veins also tend to fade after pregnancy. Reassess your skin type during this time and rigorously use the appropriate skincare.

You may find you sweat more but this will disappear after pregnancy. Meanwhile a daily bath or shower, followed by dustings of talcum powder, will help keep you comfortable.

Hair. Often the hair becomes lank and greasy. Perms don't usually react well but hair can take most colour. Try a weekly special treatment hair conditioner (ask your hairdresser) from the third to eighth month. This will help keep hair controllable now and speed recovery afterwards. Leave conditioners on for an hour.

Nails may become brittle, ridged or damaged. Manicure and

condition them regularly, keeping them fairly short to avoid more damage. Use a strengthening nail polish, nail hardener or base coat.

Teeth. All dentists say teeth are more vulnerable during pregnancy. Morning sickness leaves acid in the mouth which can erode tooth enamel. The answer is to drink some milk or rinse with water afterwards, but don't brush for at least an hour as the tooth surface is softened and you could scratch it. Brush and floss your teeth regularly and go to your dentist at least twice during the nine months. No dentist will give X rays or anaesthetic, unless necessary, and beware of taking some antibiotics such as tetracycline, which can turn your baby's teeth yellow. Dentistry during pregnancy is free under the NHS; ask your dentist for the right form to complete.

Breasts. To prevent as much damage from stretched skin as possible, your breasts will need more support as pregnancy develops. Invest in a maternity bra. You may feel more comfortable if you wear it in bed, too. Nursing pads may be necessary for seeping milk near delivery. Strengthen muscles supporting breasts by specific exercises (see Breasts section).

Legs. Maternity support tights ease aching legs and varicose veins. Avoid high heels and rest legs (with feet up) as often as possible. Combat cramp by rubbing the area, exercising legs or bending foot backwards.

Backache. As your bump gets bigger, learn to pull yourself up and in with your shoulders down and relaxed, to avoid bad posture, backache and strained abdominal muscles.

Swelling (oedema). This is common in many women, usually in the legs, and is a result of increased pressure from the baby. Your doctor may do tests; otherwise the best cure is to lie down, legs higher than hips.

Headaches. High blood pressure could be the cause, if they occur later in pregnancy. Consult your doctor.

Indigestion and heartburn. Eat little and often (but not too close to bedtime), avoiding the foods you recognise give you indigestion. Sit up straight or sleep propped up with a pillow. Sipping a glass of milk may help.

Cosmetic surgery

Sometimes called aesthetic, corrective or plastic surgery, cosmetic surgery can correct deformities from birth (hare lips, deformed noses), disguise skin marking (scars, birthmarks), repair after accident damage, change a feature you don't like (a long or bumpy nose) or counteract the effects of ageing skin (facelifts, eyelifts). More and more women (and men, too) are now using cosmetic surgery to look better. Of course, accident damage and deformities from birth need individual specialist advice. But if you are thinking of corrective surgery to transform a part of your body that *is* in good working order or wish to rid yourself of some of the signs of ageing, here is a guide to help you.

First of all consider the ten most common queries on cosmetic surgery, to see if you're a suitable candidate. They are answered by a top NHS consultant plastic surgeon:

WHO IS SUITABLE?

Generally, anyone in good health who feels strongly enough about their appearance. Those who are unrealistic about the results, or who are doing it for someone other than themselves, aren't suitable (for instance, it won't mend a shaky marriage). I'd also be worried about carrying out cosmetic surgery on a depressed patient.

HOW DO I GO ABOUT IT?

First and foremost ask your GP for referral to a plastic surgeon. If s/he isn't sympathetic, ask to see another doctor in the practice. If you feel that they're both unsympathetic, then you *can* change your GP. Only go directly to a plastic surgeon who has been personally recommended to you by a previous patient. A list of 'reputable' plastic surgeons is available to GPs from the British Association of Aesthetic Plastic Surgeons, c/o The Royal College of Surgeons, 35–43 Lincoln's Inn Fields, London WC2A 3PN. Before surgery, always make sure that you've talked to a trained plastic surgeon (with FRCS after his or her name). Also ask where s/he has worked, which hospitals and so on, and make sure that s/he gives you all the facts, including the costs, *before* you make a decision. Some local NHS plastic surgeons will see people without a letter from their GP (your local hospital will give the consultant's name). But most will let your GP know that they've seen you.

DOES IT HURT?

It depends on what is being done and the pain threshold of the patient. Face lifts and chemical peeling are painful. Eyelids and noses can be uncomfortable but surprisingly pain-free, whereas the lip area seems to be more painful. Discuss this with your surgeon.

IS IT DANGEROUS?

Any operation is potentially dangerous. And even the most brilliant surgeons and anaesthetists have made mistakes. There is an element of risk in cosmetic surgery, but not a big one. Those with horror stories are a small minority compared to satisfied patients.

WILL IT CHANGE MY LIFE?

Maybe. It depends how you feel about it. Eyelid surgery (blepharoplasty) and collagen implants often just make you look better and less tired. Scars can never be completely erased. Nose surgery (rhinoplasty) seems to make the most difference to people. Cosmetic surgery won't change circumstances but usually bucks up self-confidence.

SHOULD I TELL ANYONE?

People usually get depressed after surgery, when the attention and build-up is over. And initial swelling, scars or black eyes can make you wonder if it was worth it. So it's wise to talk it over with at least one person.

SUPPOSING IT GOES WRONG

You should be given information about common complications, and the likely outcome of your operation, before you make your decision. A good doctor should admit it if something has gone wrong and nurse the patient through their disappointment, while offering them secondary surgery at a later date. Sometimes you need touch up procedures; on noses, for example. If you're unhappy with cosmetic surgery after the swelling has gone down, you should return to your surgeon and discuss it. Most want happy, satisfied patients and so will do what they possibly can to get them. Many surgeons will recommend a second opinion if they don't agree that something went wrong. If you are still dissatisfied, the only alternative is to see a solicitor with a view to legal action. But proving negligence is expensive, difficult and takes a long time.

WHAT AGE AND STAGE IS BEST FOR COSMETIC SURGERY?

It depends on what is being corrected. Noses can be done at any time after puberty. Eyelid correction, if it's hereditary, from about 20 onwards. After 40 is the right time for cosmetic treatment related to ageing (eyelid correction, collagen for wrinkles, etc). But it's best to get individual, informed opinion from a plastic surgeon.

WHAT'S AVAILABLE ON THE NHS?

Not collagen injections except, in rare cases, for scars and burns. Almost everything else *can* be, depending on the availability of resources. Doctors will usually recommend cosmetic surgery on the NHS if the problem causes anguish and mental stress or if there's a functional problem, such as interference with vision or a blocked nose.

WHY DO WE HEAR MORE ABOUT COSMETIC SURGERY IN THE USA?

Society there has decided that beauty is a right and equals success and happiness. Here, fewer talk about it but 'ordinary people', rather than just the rich or famous, are now undergoing cosmetic surgery. Costs vary enormously but you may equate corrective surgery to the price of a family holiday and it lasts a lot longer.

Below are outlined the most usual cosmetic surgery procedures:

NOSE SURGERY (Rhinoplasty)

Who is suitable? Any fit and healthy adult with realistic expectations.

Time: 20–30 minutes' consultation; one-hour operation; at least one night in hospital. Plaster comes off seven days later. Check-up three months later.

Approximate cost: It varies, but around £1,500 for the total package. It may be available on the NHS but there are long waiting lists.

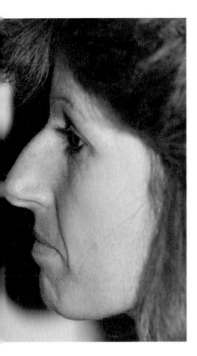

Time for face to return to normal: The bruising and swelling go down over two weeks. The new nose shape takes up to six months to settle.

Drawbacks: One in twenty patients need a secondary touch-up operation. You'll need two weeks out of circulation.

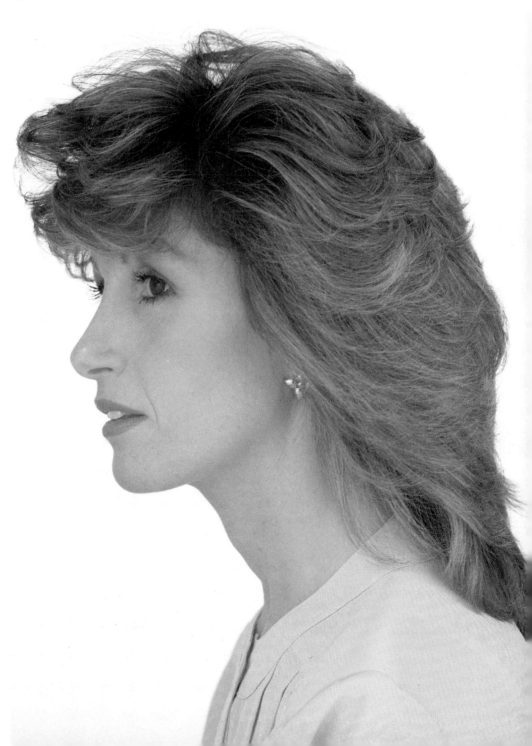

COLLAGEN IMPLANTS

Zyderm is collagen from cowhide in a salt, water and local anaesthetic solution. It is injected by a skilled doctor, along wrinkle lines at small intervals, to form a ridge and then it evens out the line as the water content of the zyderm is absorbed, lifting up the wrinkle indentation.

Who is suitable? Those with wrinkles, acne pits or depressed scars.

Time: A half-hour consultation and half an hour for each syringe treatment (three sessions, every other week). Check-up is two weeks later.

Approximate cost: £60 for the consultation and allergy test, £200 per syringe. So £660 for the first course and £200 for a top-up. But prices may vary.

Time for face to return to normal: Slight swelling is visible for a couple of hours to a few days later and needle pricks are visible for a day or so.

Drawbacks: An allergy to the collagen. On-going costs (top-ups are needed every six to twelve months).

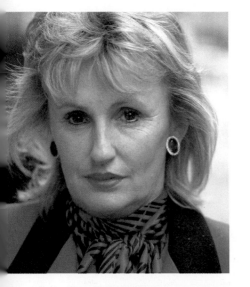

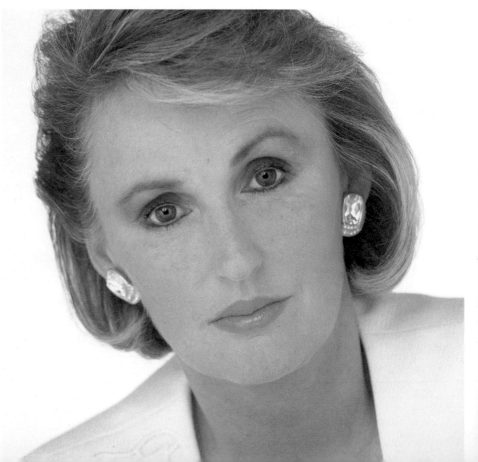

EYE LIFTS
(Blepharophryplasty)

Eye bags are either hereditary or caused by increasing age. Cosmetic surgeons advise treating hereditary eye bags early in life, as the skin becomes even less elastic and stretched with age. The operation can take place as an outpatient, under local anaesthetic and sedatives, or under general anaesthetic with one or more nights' stay in hospital.

Who is suitable? Those with bags under the eyes or drooping brows. People with eye diseases should get the all clear from an ophthalmic surgeon first.

Time: A half-hour consultation, one-hour operation, 48 hours' rest. Stitches are removed four days later. Check-up is three months later.

Approximate cost: £1,000 (for the total package). The consultation alone costs up to £50. Prices do vary.

Time for face to return to normal: It takes two weeks for the bruising and black eyes to disappear and twelve weeks for the redness of scars around the eyes to look normal without make-up.

Drawback: You need two weeks out of circulation.

BREASTS

In breast *augmentation* (lifting and enlarging) sacs of silicone are inserted beneath the skin or muscles of the breasts and attached to the breast wall. Breast *reduction* is where incisions are made around the nipple and in an upside-down T-shape (under the breasts and vertically up to the nipple to resite it). Tissue is removed and the skin shaped, then resewn. The nipple is always resited and can take up to a year to settle in a permanent position.

Who is suitable? The NHS will consider you if your GP feels that you are being affected physically or psychologically by the size of your breasts. You need to be fit and have realistic expectations.

Time: Hospital stay is usually one day for augmentation and two to four nights for reduction. Stitches are removed five to ten days later.

Approximate cost: £1,500 for augmentation and £1,500 to £2,000 for reduction. Waiting lists for NHS treatment are long.

Time for breasts to return to normal: It takes three weeks, or more, for the swelling and bruising to go. Up to a year for a resited nipple to settle. The scars will fade but never disappear completely.

Drawback: Not a 100 per cent success rate. Breast surgery may affect breast feeding or nipple sensation; ask your surgeon. The surround to the prosthesis hardens in around 50 per cent of women who have breast augmentation and around 10 per cent need further treatment.

LIPOSUCTION

A small puncture is made in the skin and fat is then suctioned from the area. Most popular sites for liposuction on the body are the hips, ankles, stomach and under the chin to firm up a jawline (often in conjunction with a face lift). It is usually performed under general anaesthetic. Cost, recovery time and bruising depend on the area 'suctioned'.

Other aesthetic operations which are available:

BROW LIFT

This is not suitable for patients who have a receding hairline or thin forehead hair. It aims to smooth out creases in the forehead and to lift droopy eyebrows. Usually under general anaesthetic, a flap of skin is removed and stitched from ear to ear around the top hairline. Stitches are usually removed after fourteen days but forehead and scalp numbness at the scar area can go on for six to twelve months. Approximate cost is £1,000 to £1,250.

CHEEK AND CHIN IMPLANTS

Silicone implants can augment weak or deformed cheekbones or chins. Each require two weeks out of circulation and take around three months for swelling to go completely. Occasionally they slip or become infected (around one in 20) and need further treatment. Approximate cost is £750.

LIPS

A tuck can be made at the cupid bow of the top lip to help eliminate wrinkles and firm up the lipline. Chemical peeling or dermabrasion on the upper lip will also reduce wrinkling. The outline colour can be strengthened by tattooing your natural lipshade colour around the outline (go to an expert aesthetic surgeon, never a tattooist). Fullness can be added to ageing lips by zyplast (a harder type of zyderm) implant.

EARS

Prominent ears can be pinned back cosmetically and this operation is often done for children. Under local or general anaesthetic, a cut is made at the back of the ear and then resewn. Head bandages must be kept on for ten days but stitches may be dissolvable. The approximate cost is £750, although it's more for general anaesthetic and a hospital stay.

FACE LIFT

This is performed under local or general anaesthetic. Skin is lifted from the face, remoulded, then tucked and stitched round the hairline. The hospital stay can be as little as one day; but bandages are kept on for two or three days and complete rest is necessary for longer. Some stitches are removed after a few days and the rest after a week. The swelling and bruising last for ten to fourteen days, but numbness and tightness may remain for up to three months. Scars around the hairline fade gradually but never go completely. Face lifts are not permanent (unlike rhinoplasty), as skin loses further elasticity with age. The length of time before a secondary lift is needed varies. Facelifts cannot perform miracles, as it's the individual bone structure that decides the final aesthetic look. Approximate cost is £2,000.

LOOSE SKIN

Sagging skin on older wrinkled hands or on the body after dramatic weight loss or loss of elasticity due to pregnancy can be 'tucked'. Success and visibility of the scars depend on the area where the tuck is needed.

DERMABRASION

This is a kind of sand blasting for skin! It's most successful on facial skin, and removes the top layers where skin is scarred, pitted by spot marks, finely wrinkled or colour marked by tattoo or pigmentation age spots. Performed under local or general anaesthetic, the area treated is then bandaged for 24 hours. Make-up can cover discoloured skin after ten days and complexion will fade to its normal colour within twelve weeks. Dermabrasion does not tighten loose skin but aims to make the skin's texture better. Approximate cost is £750.

CHEMICAL PEELING

A painful process often performed after a face lift. An acid solution is applied under general anaesthetic to burn off the top layer of skin. It is suitable for restoring a youthful glow to the skin and taking away most fine wrinkles and scar and pigment patches. But chemical peeling won't improve 'pits', deep lines or enlarged pores. If skin has been covered, this is removed 24 to 48 hours later. Scabs take up to fourteen days to fall off. Discolouration of the skin fades after three to 14 weeks and skin must be protected from sun for up to 16 weeks. Improvement in the skin's look can last from one to 10 years, depending on the skin type. The hospital stay is two to three days, and the approximate cost is £750, depending on hospital stay.

BEFORE YOU DECIDE . . .

Ask your friends what they think about the idea and to give you an honest opinion; they may be afraid of upsetting your feelings. Family members may not be so objective, even feel offended if they have inherited the same characteristics (for example, a big nose). If everyone you talk to advises you against cosmetic surgery, perhaps you're being over-sensitive about something that adds character to your looks? It may stem from lack of self-confidence. Some people even develop a phobia about some aspect of their appearance and cosmetic surgery is not the way to cure it.

However, if you are sure that your lack of confidence is due to something like large breasts or bags under your eyes, cosmetic surgery can make a large difference to your life. But do not expect it to change your lifestyle. For instance, it won't make you more attractive to men or help you to get a new job. In fact, some of the best cosmetic surgery often goes unnoticed by the nearest and dearest of those who've changed their looks. People may just say 'You look well' or 'Have you been on holiday?' so don't expect a dramatic reaction.

Think long and hard about your reasons and talk over all the possible options and side-effects with your surgeon. A cosmetic surgeon should not pressurise you into setting a date, but allow you as long as you need to think about it. S/he should also be prepared to talk it over in several consultations (which you will be asked to pay for) if you feel it's necessary.

CHAPTER 10

Calm and Collected

Complete your good looks and give beauty maximum power by
working on a healthy disposition. Inside beauty comes from learning
how to control stress and use it to your advantage, how to relax and
get a good night's sleep for reserves of calm and energy. Or you can
soothe and stimulate the mind and body by exercise or massage
techniques – done at home or taught by an expert at a beauty salon,
health club or gym. All these take time and effort to achieve, but
the rewards are well worth it.

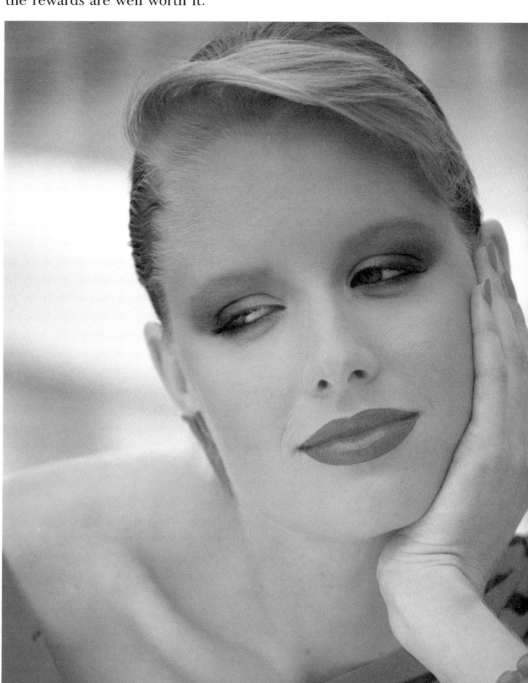

Stress

We all need some stress in our lives. The hormones adrenalin and noradrenalin are produced in response to stress and are part of our survival mechanism, gearing up our systems for fight or flight in times of danger when survival of the fittest was paramount. These days we rarely face the same kind of life and death situations and healthy tension gets us going about our daily chores, motivates us into doing larger tasks and revs up the system to face physical demands.

But too much stress can have disastrous effects on our health and well being. It can raise blood pressure and cholesterol levels leading to heart disease, tighten muscles causing pain such as headaches, lower resistance to disease, cause insomnia, ulcers and generally run down and overwork the body's system. Side effects are symptoms such as falling hair, bad skin and lack of energy. Our family, friends and colleagues suffer, too: we become irritable, temperamental, aggressive and misjudge decisions.

SIGNS OF STRESS

Watch out for these in yourself and others: anxiety, depression, overreaction, constant tiredness, short temper, insomnia, headaches, lack of energy, bad memory, over drinking and smoking, breathlessness, digestive troubles, boredom, fearfulness, phobia and suspicion. At worst stress can lead to blackouts, deep depression, mental breakdown and thoughts of suicide.

HOW NOT TO COPE WITH STRESS

The worst mistakes are made by trying to find artificial supports to remove the symptoms of stress: drinking or eating to excess, smoking or taking drugs (including tranquillisers or sleeping pills). Whilst doctors do prescribe drugs to stop tension or help sleep, these are temporary measures and should be reserved for those who are trying to cope with deep tragedy or a stressful situation that will pass. They will not alleviate the cause nor allow you to cope with on-going stress. And some doctors believe that these drugs interfere with the grieving process in any tragedy and don't allow the patient to cope with the problem realistically. Tranquillisers and sleeping pills calm you down while anti-depressants liven you up, take longer to work and need to be prescribed at exactly the right dose to do you good. They can have unpleasant side effects, especially if you suddenly stop taking them. If they are prescribed for you, check with your doctor about side effects, how long you should take them for, how they react with other drugs (the Pill, antihistamine) and whether you can drink and drive whilst under their effects.

SO HOW SHOULD YOU COPE?

Finding the cause and removing it is the simplest way, but situations over which you have no control can cause the most stress. And it varies between individuals. A day with nothing to do may seem like a complete luxury to you, while another may be severely frustrated by the boredom of unplanned time. Some love the idea of parachuting or hang-gliding, others feel sick at the thought of them. Some may find a nine to five job repetitive and tedious whilst another may love the security of regular hours. So you must assess what stresses you and how much you can take before feeling under severe pressure, to avoid it where possible. If you're not sure why, but feeling stressed, write down all the problems you have, if possible when they arise. At the same time write down achievements and successes to see what is going right and perhaps help you to cope with the problem areas. Then work out how to dispel the causes of stress.

Some stressful situations can't be changed, and as everyone suffers at some time, it's worth learning how to relax and calm down. The way you ease tension or calm down varies between individuals and so you need to find your particular tension breaker: exercise gets rid of built-up tension physically, so swimming or a long walk in fresh air may help when you feel uptight. You may find punching a cushion, moaning to a sympathetic friend, baking a cake, giving yourself a treat or day dreaming is the release you need. Otherwise try one of the easing tension treatments or exercises below. But remember not to ignore feelings of stress and to do something constructive about them when they occur.

Cut down stress by using the appropriate reaction when you feel under pressure:

Release anger if you think it's right for the situation. Or take yourself away from the situation and curse or shout in private. Be constructive and use pent-up energy to do household chores.

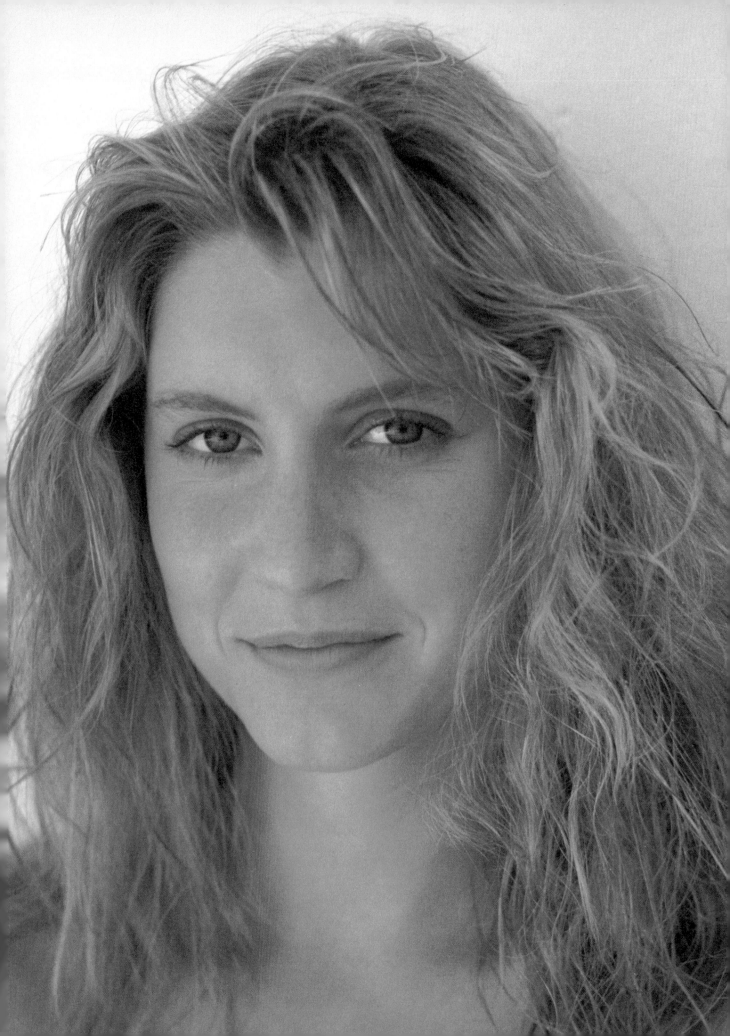

Find a haven, a room or park where you can be quiet, undisturbed and calm to control anger and stress. Feel yourself relaxing and gaining control again.

Be positive. Try to turn a frustrating situation to your advantage (for example, a spell in hospital to catch up on reading, a missed train time to do some shopping).

Be kind to yourself. In a rigid schedule allow yourself a treat occasionally when you feel you have achieved something (an evening out when working hard, a new lipstick after a failed job interview, a cup of coffee after you've written those letters and so on).

Learn to say no and mean it. Don't get yourself into disagreeable situations because you're afraid of upsetting others.

Plan ahead. Be organised to cut down stress from rush and hurrying a job.

Take support from others. Allow yourself to be helped, if you feel you can't cope.

Avoid:

Drinking over two units of alcohol a day (two pub measures of spirits, 2 glasses of wine or 1 pint of beer).

Prolonged use of tranquillisers, anti-depressants or sleeping tablets. You can become addicted.

Smoking. It causes more stress to the system.

Overeating. Too much food won't solve the problem and may add to it, if you become overweight. A balanced diet helps keep the body healthy to fight 'bad' nerves.

Easing tension

There are some simple ways of easing tension which take a few minutes and can be of benefit during a busy day or to relax before you go to bed. The easiest one is to have a warm bath after a bout of strenuous activity (and this can mean anything from cleaning out cupboards to more structured exercises). But don't suddenly spur tense muscles into action, they're liable to damage more easily. Before energetic exercise, or in some spare time during the day, try these to reduce tension:

Correct posture. It's the basis of all relaxation techniques. (See the posture section in Chapter 6.)

Breathe correctly. Sitting in the best posture position with back straight and shoulders down and relaxed, take five slow deep breaths. Now breathe in slowly to a count of three, expanding the chest as you do so. Try not to show effort or for this breathing to be noticeable to others (so you can do this one anywhere; you don't expand lungs fully and it feels 'easy' rather than forced). Now breathe out to a mental count of three. Keep up this rhythm for a minute or.so every five to 10 minutes, and use it (in traffic jams, interviews, whenever you feel nervous but aren't talking) to calm you down. Practise breathing like this at other times, when you aren't stressed.

At home in bed lie with low cushions under your head and knees. Place your palms flat on your stomach with fingertips touching. Expand your stomach as you breathe in to a count of three and feel your fingertips separating. Allow fingers to gently push down on your stomach as you breathe out again to a count of three.

Stretch. While lying, start clenching each section of your body in turn, from the tips of your toes gradually up to your head. Then relax each section in turn. Or standing, gradually stretch your body as high and rigidly as you comfortably can, so that you end up with your hands above your head and on tiptoe. Now gradually relax until you're like a limp rag doll. Do these several times until you feel relaxed.

Circle. Breathing regularly and easily, allow your head to drop forwards with chin on chest. Now start the circle slowly by moving your head to the left so that it's resting on your shoulder, then as far back as it will go. Continue the circle round to your right shoulder then back to your chest. Do the same with each shoulder, making circles in the air with the tip of your shoulder; this will ease neck and back tension. You can make circles in the air with hands, arms, legs and feet to ease joints there, too.

Mind relaxation. Clear your mind from worries and pressures with an exercise designed to relax it. Close your eyes and imagine a pleasant peaceful scene. It may be one that you already know or an imagined one . . . perhaps rolling green countryside on a spring day or an idyllic white beach in sunshine. Try to hear the sounds (birds/leaves in the wind/lapping waves) and smell the scents (grass/flowers/suncream/salt/barbecue). Now put yourself in that scene, perhaps taking a gentle walk or sitting on the beach. Try to notice all that's around you: the blue sky, the feel of sand between your toes, the warmth of the sun. A few minutes' daydreaming will relax and refresh you, allow you to clear your mind and cope with stress more easily.

Beauty treatments to relax and refresh

Here are some exercises or treatments which will help to calm you down and tone you up.

Yoga. The most popular and easiest starting point to yoga is hatha yoga with exercises designed to strengthen, flex and define the body as well as relax and refresh the mind. The aim is to perform them with as much grace and control as possible, so a sense of achievement and inner peace is developed, too. You need an expert teacher to learn how to practise yoga and should let them know if you're pregnant or have back, heart or any other health problem. Before you join a yoga class, make sure you haven't eaten for at least an hour or two; wear comfortable, flexible clothing and you may need a blanket or mat to work on. Between sessions try to practise every day.

Massage. By applying pressure to parts of the body you can help blood flow more easily and so deliver oxygen and nutrients to organs of the body while eliminating waste products quicker. It will also

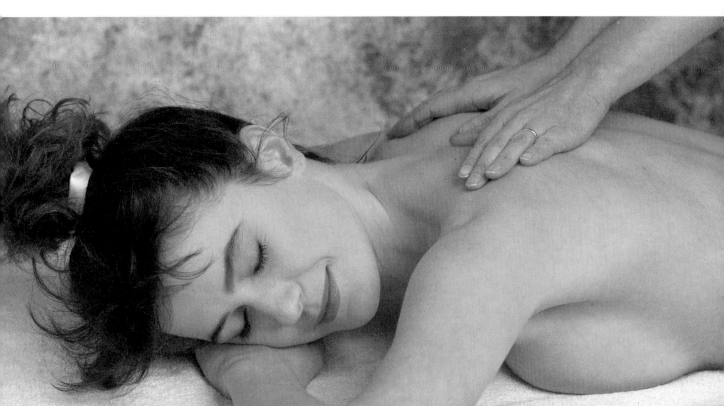

push tense muscles back into shape and so stop aches and allow better blood supply. Massage should never be done on those suffering from high blood pressure, thrombosis, varicose veins, recent injuries or skin complaints. A masseur at a health club should look clean and have short nails.

Massage should be done with the finger pads, palms or sides of the hands, using oil. Stroking, kneading, tapping and chopping motions are used. The safest one for the inexperienced, who may be massaging a partner, is the stroking movement. At home, try these on yourself or your partner, going gently at first and always stopping if the recipient feels any ache or pain.

For the face, using the fingertips of both hands, stroke from nose bridge out over brows at mid temple to outer brow, round at temples, around cheekbones to nose. Then from below ear round and up jaw to chin.

For back and shoulders, with partner lying face down or sitting, start stroking with fingertips of both hands at mid back just below nape of neck going up and round to shoulders. In one sweeping movement each time, start lower and reach further along shoulders until you go from small of back to shoulder tips. Gently pinch area between shoulderbone and neck and gently knead with thumbs base of neck up to skull bone.

Aromatherapy uses specially scented oils with massage to revive, refresh, relax or relieve you. Claims of relieving rheumatism, insomnia, loss of libido, sinus problems and many more ills are made by aromatherapists. It's best to allow a few hours after treatment to relax and give the oils time to sink in (four to six hours) before you wash.

Acupuncture needles are inserted along what the ancient Orientals believed were energy channels in the body. Some modern doctors believe that these points are connected with the nervous system and that the needles block pain messages to the brain. Acupuncturists claim to relieve stress, cure aches and pain, improve skin, stop you smoking and so on. Whether you believe the physiology or not, alternative medicine including acupuncture is popular and has certainly helped some sufferers. Remember to check that the needles have been thoroughly sterilised before allowing operation to commence.

Shiatsu or Acupressure uses the acupuncture points but instead of inserting needles, pressure is applied to these energy points to ease aches, pains, tension and fatigue. Unlike other massages, the giver uses different parts of their body as well as their hands to apply pressure (there is no stroking or kneading, simply pressure and stretching) and benefits are supposedly felt by both parties.

Hypnosis or auto-suggestive programmes can teach you to relax, usually by rhythmic suggestion. Some of us are supposedly more susceptible to hypnosis than others; some hypnotists are supposedly better than others.

Exercise for the mind also includes ancient Oriental arts which require greater application and time to learn. The basic yoga exercises can be practised easily, whereas T'ai-Chi, Alexander Technique, kendo, judo and karate need expert tuition and hours of study before you'll become proficient.

T'ai-Chi Ch'uan requires minimum muscle contraction and a relaxed but positive attitude. It's a type of slow fluid dance routine that you do on your own, with controlled movements involving meditation.

The Alexander Technique or Principle involves exercises to balance and become aware of how your body works, applying your mind to get the best from your physique. It emphasises stretching the spine and holding the head at a proper angle, so is ideal for backache sufferers.

Kendo, Judo and Karate are survival and fighting exercises which include interaction with a partner. Based on balance and control they involve fast precise movements. These sports are now played mainly for combat expertise and the confidence of knowing how to protect yourself, if necessary. Judo is particularly suitable for women who feel anxious about being able to defend themselves, as the movements rely on balance rather than sheer body mass to floor a potential attacker. They all help to tone and define the body, relieve stress and create self-confidence.

Sleep

It's not for nothing that sleep is called 'beauty' sleep. Sleep restores and recharges the body. It alleviates mental fatigue and reinforces the immune system to fight off infection and illness. That is why it's so important to sleep when you're ill or run down and also why you feel tired at these times. Sleep is an excellent treatment for stress and it helps clear the mind, allowing you to see things more realistically on awakening.

We spend around a third of our lifetime unconscious, in sleep. But requirements differ for individuals. Some exist happily on four hours a night, while others need at least ten to feel in top form. How long you sleep changes as you get older. Newborn babies need 14 to 18 hours to help them mature, but by the time they reach fifty the average is around seven hours a day. Pregnant women need a couple of hours more, pre-menstrually women often require more sleeping hours and the newly bereaved also appear to sleep for longer. But the hours of quality sleep are more important than overall time. During the first hour to an hour and a half of quiet (slow wave) sleep, we slow down and bodily temperature drops. This is followed by a gradual dropping into deeper sleep, called 'rapid eye movement' or REM sleep, in which the brain becomes active, the eyes dart from side to side under usually-closed lids, as you dream. Everyone dreams, women more than men, even if they don't remember it in the morning. Usually only those woken abruptly by a loud noise, movement or the dream itself (nightmare) remember their dreams clearly. Whether these dreams serve any useful purpose to our waking lives is still a case for argument. But dreams are believed to act as a kind of file for the subconscious, to work through past and present experiences and allow them to be stored. REM sleep is, therefore, useful as a sort of mental therapy, whereas the lighter, slow wave sleep affords the body rest, repair and recovery. Lack of sleep can cause hallucinations, disorientation and, if for a prolonged time, mental disturbance.

So how much do you need? We can all miss one or even two nights' sleep without severe ill effects; even though you may feel rough and light-headed, this is due to habit and emotional needs rather than physical ones. And you can catch up on sleep. A sleepless night or week of late nights and early mornings can be restored by longer sleep at the weekend. Those who sleep easily and feel refreshed whatever their requirement of sleep are said to live for longer. So try to indulge yourself with as much sleep as you feel happy with, when you have the time.

GETTING ENOUGH

Over ten per cent of the British take sleeping pills to get their nightly slumber. But these are addictive and should only be used in extreme circumstances. Regular use also reduces the impact of these drugs. Eighty per cent of the causes of insomnia are some form of emotional upset: depression, stress, anxiety (often about not getting to sleep!) and so on. External causes such as light or noise (a new baby), keep the other 20 per cent of insomniacs awake. Doctors now believe that around five hours' sleep a night is the healthy minimum for the average adult. If you have difficulty in sleeping, try these tips:

Write a list of all the things you need to do the next day or the worries on your mind. Exercise about an hour before going to bed, follow this with a warm bath and a small portion of a carbohydrate-type food (bread, apple juice, figs). Then settle down with a jigsaw or an easygoing (not too exciting) book. Sex, when you feel like it, can give more contented sleep.

Avoid tea, coffee, sugar and salty foods as well as smoking and larger meals just before retiring. Tea, coffee, sugar and salt are stimulants and help wake you up. Smoking produces a chemical which hinders sleep. And your digestive system slows down during the night and won't be able to break down large meals so easily, so they'll lie heavily on the stomach. A thimbleful of alcohol (brandy) can help relax you if you're still feeling energetic but tired at the end of a long day. But never take more, as too much alcohol will keep you awake and disturb deep sleep during the night.

Make sure your bedroom is warm and well aired. Try to reduce noise and light to a minimum, perhaps by changing to a back room away from road traffic and getting heavier, more dense curtains to shut out light. Partners who snore or move around when they're asleep are a problem. It's up to you to decide whether the togetherness of a double bed or the same room is worth less ease in sleeping.

Make sure your bed suits you. You need a mattress at least nine inches longer than your length. Make sure it is firm enough to support you and soft enough to mould round curves (you should not be able to fit your hand between mattress and the small of your back when you are lying on it). Make sure you get a wide enough bed if you and your partner both spread out during the night. And find one where two mattresses are joined in a single frame if you vary dramatically in size or weight. Mattresses wear out and don't give enough support after ten years or so; change yours for a new one for easy relaxed sleep. Don't sleep on two pillows, which can hinder breathing, instead go for a flatter type which supports but moulds to your head. Duvets take on your own shape and so help prevent draughts cooling you down too much during the night. But blankets can be anchored more easily for restless sleepers.

- If you still can't sleep, try counting sheep. Boring, repetitive mental exercises help the mind to switch off. If all else fails, get up and do some strenuous exercises (dust the pelmets, wash the walls) before trying some more relaxing, restful exercises, such as the daydreaming as mentioned in the Easing Tension section.

IF YOU SUFFER FROM INSOMNIA

- Do take plenty of physical exercise during the day. Try to play tennis or go swimming in the early evening and don't relax too much afterwards; play a game of chess or do a crossword rather than dozing in front of the TV until it's time for bed.
- Don't nap during the day. Allow yourself to get tired.
- Don't go to bed until you're tired and then make sure it's during night hours.
- Don't oversleep in the morning. Get up earlier if you have trouble getting to sleep at night.
- Make sure your bedroom is a restful environment. Don't allow any work into the room.
- Don't worry about lack of sleep. If your body needs sleep desperately, it will get it as soon as you allow yourself to relax.
- You may like to try hypnotherapy for instruction on self-hypnosis – a way of relaxing the body to get it ready for the first stage of sleep. (See Hypnosis section.)

Energy

This is the 'collected' part of the title of this chapter. To collect energy and produce adrenalin you first need to make sure the body is well fuelled with food (calories are units of energy; other nutrients in food help them work in the body) and oxygen. These, combined with stimulus motivation from the brain, react chemically to spur the body into action when we need it.

You can read about fuelling the body in Chapter 6. And oxygen is available to all of us, through air. But what causes motivation? If you're lucky it can be triggered by a sunny day, a kind word or

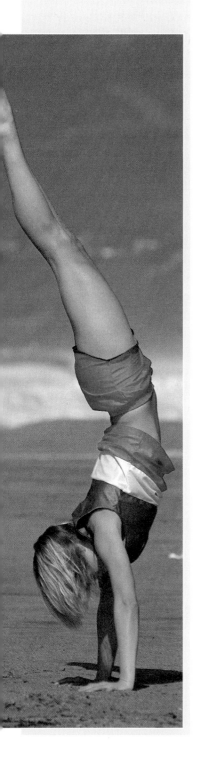

elevating news. Or you can set your own motivation and achievement goals. Experts suggest you should make both short and long term goals. They should be easy to achieve, realistic, ongoing and rewarding (to yourself or through those around you). And you should record them (in a diary) for feedback.

Fortunately, using energy can create more energy. Exercise expends energy, but rather than sapping strength, it tends to help motivation, increase air consumption (and therefore oxygen) and create hunger. Exercise also uses these energy boosters to their best advantage, directing food and oxygen to the muscles and (a left-over from our cave dwelling ancestors) making the body work in the way for which it was originally designed – physically as well as mentally. One of the magical ingredients of energy can inspire demand for another. Fresh unpolluted air also creates hunger and can liven us

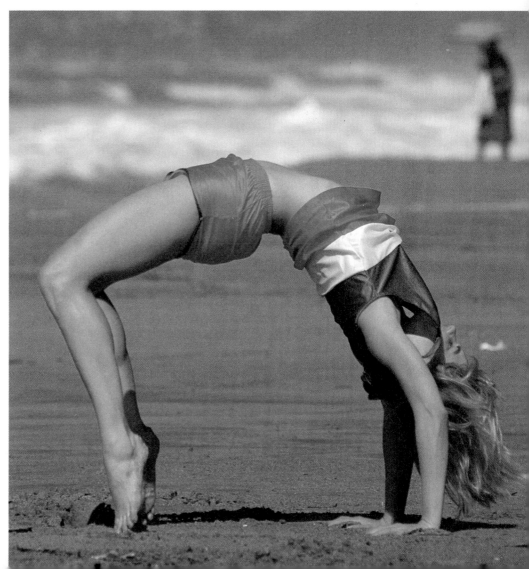

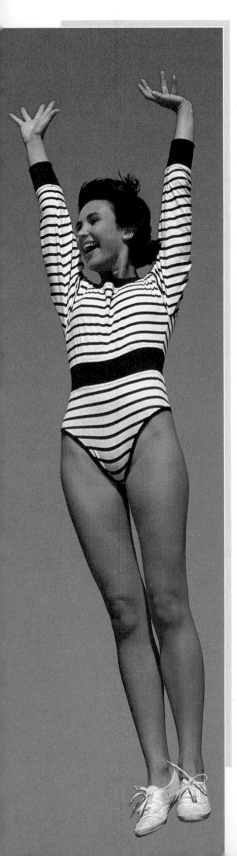

up; for example, going for a walk in the oxygen-intensive countryside or by the sea shore wakes us up. Food takes longer to work because it needs to break down and be digested by our systems before entering our bloodstream and giving goodness where it's needed. But ask anyone who has been 'off' food for a few days how they feel after satisfying their hunger with a good meal and it will usually be more 'alive'. Being motivated by good news or achievement can increase hunger and make you feel the need for activity.

This sparking off of one ingredient against another should, by all intents, ensure that we're bouncing with energy all the time. But unfortunately a bad diet, polluted atmospheres or smoking and demotivators, such as stress, boredom, lack of sleep or depression, stop 'good' energy being produced. Instead they create a more destructive type of chemical from the adrenal gland which dampens down our system, so energy is retained in reserve for internal disorders, rather than gearing up our muscles and senses for a happier, more active time.

These will hinder energy, some more immediately than others, and are worth avoiding: alcohol, smoking, polluted atmospheres, air conditioned atmospheres, heat, too heavy meals (energy is directed towards digestion), crash diets, lack of exercise, stress, boredom, illness, and physical injury.

For continued energy, make sure that you:
- Eat properly.
- Get enough fresh air.
- Avoid or cope with stress.
- Take regular exercise.

For a daily energy boost, try these tips:
- Do 15 minutes of exercise on waking.
- Eat breakfast; it releases energy gradually during the day.
- Avoid alcohol at lunchtime but eat a light lunch of fresh or raw vegetables with some protein food such as fish, eggs or lean meat.
- Give yourself regular treats and incentives after you've achieved something – it may be as simple as watching the television or a phone call to a favourite friend after finishing a good number of chores.
- Walk whenever you can.

Beauty and the Beast

There is simply no point in trying to look your best when you're miserable inside. Clinical depression is very different from the blue moods that occur when your life isn't running smoothly, and those suffering from serious prolonged depression should see their doctor for advice. But if you feel your life just isn't as fulfilled and happy as it might be, this will certainly show up in, and hinder, your looks, usually in the form of frown lines and bad posture.

It's been proved that people who take care of their looks, and also appear happy, are seen as more bright and attractive to others. So if you suspect your life could do with some changes, now is the time to work them out.

How? Reassess your lifestyle; you may find by moving homes, changing jobs or making new friends, your lifestyle becomes more interesting and enjoyable. It may mean grasping confidence with both hands and joining a club or evening class in something which interests you and where you'll meet new people. Or resolving not to see over-critical friends who make you feel unhappy about yourself. If a situation which is depressing you can't be changed, try to alter the rules a little; for example, arrange more time to yourself if you are too much at home with elderly relatives or troublesome teenagers. Be constructive about a failing relationship at home or work and try to sort it out in some way. If financial problems are making you feel insecure, see your bank manager for advice on budgeting for regular payments; make sure basic insurance covers are paid and perhaps take a part-time job if you don't work and the burden is falling on your partner to work longer hours for overtime payments. Sort out priorities. A new dress may buck up your self esteem more than a night out.

Sending your children to summer camp and spending a romantic weekend away with your partner in Britain could be a happier alternative than a two-week family holiday. Or perhaps, to you personally, getting your nose fixed by cosmetic surgery or keeping your hair a summer blond at the hairdresser's all year round take priority over a holiday.

Some careful thought and good judgement will do you and those around you a favour by making you an all-round attractive person. And remember that the best beauty bonus is a smile; you'll feel happier and appear happier – so put one on every day!

Acknowledgements

A complete beauty book would be impossible to write without the help, advice and generosity of others. I'd like to give a heartfelt thanks to the following:

Carol Johns for her untiring research and computer wizardry with the manuscript.

Dermatologist Steve Wright, MA, MRCP at the London Hospital for advice on Chapter 2.

Silvikrin, Jon Gordon, Keith at Alan & Co., Paul Edmonds for hairstyle photographs.

Dr R. C. Cottrell and Jenny Salmon, MSc, BSc, for advice on Chapter 6. Shelley Preston of Bucks Fizz for modelling the ideal figure. Sainsbury's for the food photograph.

Dentist Stephen L. Selwyn, BDS (Lond), LDSD Orth, RCS (Eng), Gillian Richards-Gray at the Optical Information Council, Plastic surgeon D. M. Davies, FRCS and Dr Alexander D. G. Gunn of Reading University Health Centre for their advice on Chapter 9.

Krissie Butcher, Mercia Watkins and the Harley Medical Group for their before-and-after cosmetic surgery photographs.

Wendy Harris for the pregnancy photograph.

Behavioural Psychotherapist Rob Newell for advice on Chapter 10. Photographer Liz McAulay for the mother and baby photograph.

For photographs throughout the book: Al Macdonald, Serge Krouglikoff, Chris Craymer, Alex James, David J. Anthony, Adrian Bradbury, Liz McAulay, Martin Evening, Colin Thomas, Rob Lee and Peter Underwood.

And last, but by no means least, those in the Beauty Department of *Woman* for their help and research: Penny Farmer and Pat Eldridge.

Index